Case Studies in
Diabetology and Endocrinology

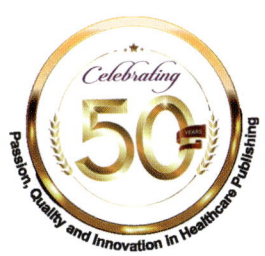

Case Studies in
Diabetology and Endocrinology

Editors

Sanjay Chatterjee Dip. BMSc MD Certificate in Diabetes Care
Honorary Consultant Diabetologist
Apollo Hospital
Kolkata, West Bengal, India

Sudip Chatterjee MD MNAMS FRCP FACP
Honorary Professor
Vivekananda Institute of Medical Sciences
Honorary Secretary
Park Clinic
Kolkata, West Bengal, India

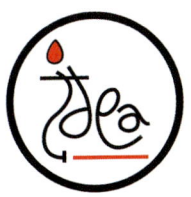

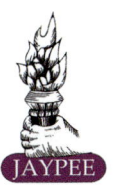

JAYPEE BROTHERS MEDICAL PUBLISHERS
The Health Sciences Publisher
New Delhi | London | Panama

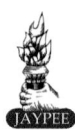 **Jaypee Brothers Medical Publishers (P) Ltd**

Headquarters
Jaypee Brothers Medical Publishers (P) Ltd
4838/24, Ansari Road, Daryaganj
New Delhi 110 002, India
Phone: +91-11-43574357
Fax: +91-11-43574314
Email: jaypee@jaypeebrothers.com

Overseas Offices

J.P. Medical Ltd
83 Victoria Street, London
SW1H 0HW (UK)
Phone: +44 20 3170 8910
Fax: +44 (0)20 3008 6180
Email: info@jpmedpub.com

Jaypee-Highlights Medical Publishers Inc
City of Knowledge, Bld. 235, 2nd Floor, Clayton
Panama City, Panama
Phone: +1 507-301-0496
Fax: +1 507-301-0499
Email: cservice@jphmedical.com

Jaypee Brothers Medical Publishers (P) Ltd
Bhotahity, Kathmandu, Nepal
Phone: +977-9741283608
Email: kathmandu@jaypeebrothers.com

Website: www.jaypeebrothers.com
Website: www.jaypeedigital.com

© 2020, Jaypee Brothers Medical Publishers

The views and opinions expressed in this book are solely those of the original contributor(s)/author(s) and do not necessarily represent those of editor(s) of the book.

All rights reserved. No part of this publication may be reproduced, stored or transmitted in any form or by any means, electronic, mechanical, photocopying, recording or otherwise, without the prior permission in writing of the publishers.

All brand names and product names used in this book are trade names, service marks, trademarks or registered trademarks of their respective owners. The publisher is not associated with any product or vendor mentioned in this book.

Medical knowledge and practice change constantly. This book is designed to provide accurate, authoritative information about the subject matter in question. However, readers are advised to check the most current information available on procedures included and check information from the manufacturer of each product to be administered, to verify the recommended dose, formula, method and duration of administration, adverse effects and contraindications. It is the responsibility of the practitioner to take all appropriate safety precautions. Neither the publisher nor the author(s)/editor(s) assume any liability for any injury and/or damage to persons or property arising from or related to use of material in this book.

This book is sold on the understanding that the publisher is not engaged in providing professional medical services. If such advice or services are required, the services of a competent medical professional should be sought.

Every effort has been made where necessary to contact holders of copyright to obtain permission to reproduce copyright material. If any have been inadvertently overlooked, the publisher will be pleased to make the necessary arrangements at the first opportunity. The **CD/DVD-ROM** (if any) provided in the sealed envelope with this book is complimentary and free of cost. **Not meant for sale.**

Inquiries for bulk sales may be solicited at: jaypee@jaypeebrothers.com

Case Studies in Diabetology and Endocrinology / Sanjay Chatterjee, Sudip Chatterjee

First Edition: **2020**

ISBN: 978-93-89188-29-5

Printed at: Samrat Offset Pvt. Ltd.

CONTRIBUTORS

EDITORS

Sanjay Chatterjee Dip. BMSc MD Certificate in Diabetes Care
Honorary Consultant Diabetologist
Apollo Hospital
Kolkata, West Bengal, India

Sudip Chatterjee MD MNAMS FRCP FACP
Honorary Professor
Vivekananda Institute of Medical Sciences
Honorary Secretary
Park Clinic
Kolkata, West Bengal, India

CONTRIBUTING AUTHORS

Ajitesh Roy MD DM
Associate Professor
Department of Endocrinology
Vivekananda Institute of Medical Sciences
Kolkata, West Bengal, India

Animesh Maiti MD DM
Associate Professor and Head
Department of Endocrinology
Medical College
Kolkata, West Bengal, India

Anirban Mazumdar MD DM FICP
Professor and Head
Department of Endocrinology
KPC Medical College and Hospital
Kolkata, West Bengal, India

Anirban Sinha MD DM FACE
Assistant Professor
Department of Endocrinology
Medical College
Kolkata, West Bengal, India

Asish Kumar Basu Dip. Card MD DM
Professor, Department of Endocrinology
Medical College
Kolkata, West Bengal, India

Binayak Sinha MBBS FRCP (Lond)
CCST Endocrinology
Consultant Endocrinologist
AMRI Hospital Salt Lake
Kolkata, West Bengal, India

Biswajit Ghoshdastidar MD MRCP
Visiting Physician
Woodlands Hospital Visiting Physician
Department of Medicine
Calcutta Medical Research Institute
Kolkata, West Bengal, India

Chandan Mishra MD
Post Doctral Trainee
Department of Endocrinology
Medical College
Kolkata, West Bengal, India

Chhavi Agrawal MD
Postdoctoral Trainee
Department of Endocrinology
Medical College
Kolkata, West Bengal, India

Chitra Selvan MD DM
Associate Professor
Department of Endocrinology
MS Ramaiah Medical College
Bengaluru, Karnataka, India

Debasis Maji MD DM
Former Head
Department of Medicine
Vivekananda Institute of Medical Sciences
Kolkata, West Bengal, India

Debmalya Sanyal DTM&H MD DM MRCP FACE
Professor
Department of Endocrinology
KPC Medical College and Hospital
Kolkata, West Bengal, India

Ghanshyam Goyal MD
Consultant Diabetologist and Diabetic Foot Specialist
ILS Hospitals, Salt Lake and SVS Marwari Hospital
Kolkata, West Bengal, India

JJ Mukherjee MD FRCP (Lond)
Senior Consultant
Division of Endocrinology
Department of Medicine
Apollo Gleneagles Hospital
Kolkata, West Bengal, India

Kalyan Kumar Gangopadhyay MD FRCP CCST
Senior Consultant in Endocrinology and Diabetes Fortis Hospital and Peerless Hospital
Kolkata, West Bengal, India

Neeraj Sinha MD DM
Assistant Professor
Department of Endocrinology
Indira Gandhi Institute of Medical Sciences
Patna, Bihar, India

Nilanjan Sengupta MD DM
Professor and Head
Department of Endocrinology
Nil Ratan Sircar Medical College
Kolkata, West Bengal, India

Partha Pratim Chakraborty MD DM DNB
RMO cum Clinical Tutor
Department of Endocrinology
Medical College
Kolkata, West Bengal, India

Partha Sarathi Choudhury MD DM
Senior Resident
Department of Endocrinology
Medical College
Kolkata, West Bengal, India

Pradip Mukhopadhyay MD DM
Associate Professor
Department of Endocrinology
IPGMER and SSKM Hospital
Kolkata, West Bengal, India

Rahin Mahata MD
Postdoctoral Trainee
Department of Endocrinology
Medical College
Kolkata, West Bengal, India

Rahul Valsaraj MD
Senior Resident
Department of Endocrinology
Nil Ratan Sircar Medical College
Kolkata, West Bengal, India

Rana Bhattacharjee MD DM MRCP FICP
Faculty, Department of Endocrinology
IPGMER and SSKM Hospital
Kolkata, West Bengal, India

Sajal Kamat MD
Senior Resident
Department of Endocrinology
Nil Ratan Sircar Medical College
Kolkata, West Bengal, India

Samit Ghosal MD MSc (Diab Care)
Consultant
Nightingale Hospital
Kolkata, West Bengal, India

Satinath Mukhopadhyay MD DM FRCP FAMS
Professor, Department of Endocrinology
Institute of Post Graduate Medical Education and Research
Kolkata, West Bengal, India

Saurav Shishir MD
Postdoctoral Trainee
Department of Endocrinology
Medical College
Kolkata, West Bengal, India

Sayan Ghosh MD
Postdoctoral Trainee
Department of Endocrinology
Medical College
Kolkata, West Bengal, India

Somnath Raghuvanshi MD
Postdoctoral Trainee
Department of Endocrinology
Medical College
Kolkata, West Bengal, India

Soumyabrata Roy Chaudhuri MSc (Diabetes)
MRCP PG Dip. Clinical Endocrinology and Diabetes
PG Certificate in Diabetes and Endocrinology
Senior Registrar
Department of Endocrinology
KPC Medical College
Kolkata, West Bengal, India

Subhankar Chowdhury DTM&H MD DM MRCP
Professor and Head
Department of Endocrinology
Institute of Post Graduate Medical Education and Research
Kolkata, West Bengal, India

Subir Ray MD FRCP (Edin)
Senior Consultant
Apollo Gleneagles Hospitals
Kolkata, West Bengal, India

Sujoy Ghosh MD DM FRCP FICP FACE
Associate Professor
Department of Endocrinology
IPGMER and SSKM Hospital
Kolkata, West Bengal, India

Sujoy Majumdar MD MRCP
FRCP (Lond, Dub)
Honorary Head
GD Hospital and Diabetes Institute
Senior Consultant Endocrinologist
Peerless Hospital and Ruby General Hospital
Kolkata, West Bengal, India

Tapas Chandra Das MD DM
MO Physician
Department of Medicine
Ranaghat SD Hospital
Ranaghat, West Bengal, India

PREFACE

In 2010, a group of physicians practicing in the fields of Diabetology and Endocrinology felt the need of forming an organization for the advancement in learning and fostering knowledge in the fields of Diabetology, Endocrinology, Metabolic Disorders and Clinical Nutrition. With that objective, the Integrated Diabetes and Endocrine Academy (IDEA) was formed in 2011. From a small and humble beginning, it grew up to become an eminent organization and its annual conference, the IDEACON has become one of the most sought after conferences in India.

The activities of IDEA include holding regular monthly CMEs, holding health camps in Kolkata and nearby villages, distributing free insulin to poor patients, holding IDEACON and supporting medical research. Another initiative of IDEA has been the publication of handbooks on diabetes, endocrinology and related disorders. Two books have been already published by eminent publishers and the books were freely distributed to IDEACON delegates in 2017 and 2018.

The earlier books were on common disorders in diabetes and endocrinology. This time, the book deals with uncommon problems in diabetes and endocrinology which a physician may face in his/her clinical practice. This is a case-based approach and the cases are all real-world cases, actually seen by the contributors. We were fortunate to get valuable contributions from IPGMER, Medical College and Nil Ratan Sircar Medical College, Kolkata, West Bengal, India, institutions where DM courses in endocrinology are conducted. We are grateful to all our authors from these institutions and to those from the IDEA fold, all of whom have freely given their time and effort to contribute to this casebook. The book covers a wide range of uncommon clinical problems or unusual clinical presentation. Sometimes the presentation is fairly common, and the authors have discussed complex management protocols.

We are grateful to Jaypee Brothers Medical Publishers (P) Ltd. for publishing the book and to Mr Sabyasachi Hazra in particular as without his constant support and follow up the book would never have taken shape. We acknowledge the support of Mr Ranandu Bhattacharya of Cipla in producing this book. All of us, authors and editors alike will feel successful, if this book serves the purpose for which it was intended and created.

Sanjay Chatterjee
Sudip Chatterjee

CONTENTS

SECTION 1: ADRENAL

CASE 1: Adrenal Histoplasmosis — 1
Tapas Chandra Das, Neeraj Sinha, Partha Sarathi Choudhury, Anirban Sinha, Animesh Maiti, Asish Kumar Basu

CASE 2: Pheochromocytoma without Hypertension — 3
Saurav Shishir, Chhavi Agrawal, Partha Sarathi Choudhury, Partha Pratim Chakraborty, Anirban Sinha, Animesh Maiti, Asish Kumar Basu

CASE 3: A 32-year-old Man with Hypertension — 5
JJ Mukherjee

CASE 4: Giddiness and Near-syncope Post Pacemaker Implantation—Not Always Cardiac or Neurogenic — 10
Soumyabrata Roy Chaudhuri

CASE 5: Triple A Syndrome — 13
Rana Bhattacharjee, Pradip Mukhopadhyay, Sujoy Ghosh

CASE 6: Evolving Primary Adrenal Insufficiency — 14
Rana Bhattacharjee, Ajitesh Roy, Pradip Mukhopadhyay, Sujoy Ghosh

SECTION 2: BONES

CASE 1: Pseudofracture (Looser's Zone) with Subsequent Low Trauma Fracture: Under-recognized but not Uncommon Presentation of Distal Renal Tubular Acidosis — 17
Subhankar Chowdhury, Partha Pratim Chakraborty

CASE 2: Refractory Rickets due to Fanconi's Syndrome Secondary to Wilson's Disease — 20
Chitra Selvan, Rana Bhattacharjee, Pradip Mukhopadhyay, Sujoy Ghosh

SECTION 3: DEVELOPMENT

CASE 1: A Short Girl with Delayed Puberty — 23
Anirban Mazumdar

SECTION 4: DIABETES

CASE 1: A Young Ketosis Prone Diabetic — 27
Anirban Mazumdar

CASE 2:	Common Problem...Where Lies the Solution? *Biswajit Ghoshdastidar*	30
CASE 3:	A Diabetic with Infected Hand *Anirban Mazumdar*	33
CASE 4:	Advanced Diabetic Nephropathy without Diabetic Retinopathy *Debmalya Sanyal*	35
CASE 5:	Diabetes Mellitus *Debasis Maji*	38
CASE 6:	Diabetes and the Breast *Kalyan Kumar Gangopadhyay*	41
CASE 7:	Cellulitis Mimic in Diabetes *Kalyan Kumar Gangopadhyay*	44
CASE 8:	Heart Failure as a Presentation of Diabetes *Nilanjan Sengupta, Sajal Kamat*	46
CASE 9:	Antihyperglycemic Agents and Hospitalization for Heart Failure: A Practical Issue *Samit Ghosal*	50
CASE 10:	Modern Management of Type 2 Diabetes Mellitus: Making Sense of the Multiple Options *Samit Ghosal*	54
CASE 11:	Approach to a Patient of Type 2 Diabetes Mellitus with Unexplained Hyperglycemic State *Sanjay Chatterjee*	57
CASE 12:	Fibrocalculus Pancreatic Diabetes Presenting as Pancreatic Adenocarcinoma *Satinath Mukhopadhyay, Partha Pratim Chakraborty*	60
CASE 13:	Myonecrosis: An Unusual Microvascular Complication of Diabetes *Satinath Mukhopadhyay, Partha Pratim Chakraborty*	63
CASE 14:	Cystic Fibrosis-related Diabetes *Satinath Mukhopadhyay, Partha Pratim Chakraborty*	66
CASE 15:	A Patient with Late Onset Diabetes in Adult *Satinath Mukhopadhyay, Partha Pratim Chakraborty*	67
CASE 16:	Double Diabetes—But Differently Double *Soumyabrata Roy Chaudhuri*	69
CASE 17:	Diabetes Mellitus as Presenting Manifestation of Acromegaly due to Growth Hormone-secreting Pituitary Macroadenoma *Subhankar Chowdhury, Partha Pratim Chakraborty*	72
CASE 18:	Diabetic Truncal Radiculoneuropathy: A Completely Reversible Form of Diabetic Neuropathy *Subhankar Chowdhury, Partha Pratim Chakraborty*	75

CASE 19:	Acute Gastric Dilatation as Presenting Manifestation of Diabetic Ketoacidosis	77
	Subhankar Chowdhury, Partha Pratim Chakraborty	
CASE 20:	A Patient where Continuous Glucose Monitoring System Helped	79
	Sudip Chatterjee	
CASE 21:	A Patient with Interesting Problems	82
	Sudip Chatterjee	

SECTION 5: DIABETIC FOOT

CASE 1:	A Case of Acute Charcot's Joint	84
	Debmalya Sanyal	
CASE 2:	A Case of Charcot Foot	86
	Ghanshyam Goyal	
CASE 3:	Ischemic Diabetic Foot	90
	Ghanshyam Goyal	
CASE 4:	A Case of Diabetic Foot Infection	93
	Ghanshyam Goyal	
CASE 5:	A Case of Neuropathic Diabetic Foot	96
	Ghanshyam Goyal	

SECTION 6: GENETICS

CASE 1:	Turner Syndrome with Hyperthyroidism	100
	Anirban Mazumdar	
CASE 2:	Hypogonadal Man with Leg Ulcers	102
	Anirban Mazumdar	
CASE 3:	An Obese Hyperactive Child	104
	Anirban Mazumdar	
CASE 4:	A Boy with Macroorchidism	107
	Anirban Mazumdar	

SECTION 7: METABOLISM

CASE 1:	Central Venous Sinus Thrombosis in a Type 2 Diabetes Mellitus Patient with Marked Hypertriglyceridemia	110
	Debmalya Sanyal	
CASE 2:	To be Taken with A Pinch of Salt	112
	Kalyan Kumar Gangopadhyay	
CASE 3:	Familial Partial Lipodystrophy Masquerading as Polycystic Ovarian Syndrome: Rare or Overlooked?	115
	Subhankar Chowdhury, Partha Pratim Chakraborty	

SECTION 8: OVARIES

CASE 1: Polycystic Ovarian Syndrome: A Common Problem — 120
Rahin Mahata, Chandan Mishra, Partha Sarathi Choudhury, Anirban Sinha, Animesh Maiti, Asish Kumar Basu

SECTION 9: PANCREAS

CASE 1: Hypoglycemia Workup — 123
Binayak Sinha

SECTION 10: PARATHYROID

CASE 1: Brown Tumor of the Lower Jaw as the First Manifestation of Primary Hyperparathyroidism: A Case Report — 127
Subir Ray

CASE 2: An Interesting Case of Acute Confusional State — 129
Sujoy Majumdar

SECTION 11: PITUITARY

CASE 1: Uncontrolled Hyperglycemia–Think beyond Glycemia — 134
Animesh Maiti, Anirban Sinha, Asish Kumar Basu, Partha Sarathi Choudhury, Saurav Shishir, Chhavi Agrawal

CASE 2: Hot Flashes in Men: Rare Presentation of a Rare Disorder — 136
Biswajit Ghoshdastidar

CASE 3: Snake and the Pituitary — 139
Kalyan Kumar Gangopadhyay

CASE 4: Prolactinoma: A Rare and Treatable Cause of Male Infertility — 142
Nilanjan Sengupta, Rahul Valsaraj

CASE 5: Secondary Hypothyroidism: Easy to Miss — 144
Sudip Chatterjee

SECTION 12: THYROID

CASE 1: Enlarged Pituitary in Primary Hypothyroidism — 146
Ajitesh Roy

CASE 2: Thyroid Ophthalmopathy — 149
Sayan Ghosh, Somnath Raghuvanshi, Partha Sarathi Choudhury, Anirban Sinha, Animesh Maiti, Asish Kumar Basu

CASE 3: Graves' Disease with Ocular Myasthenia Gravis — 151
Anirban Mazumdar

CASE 4: Gestational Thyrotoxicosis — 154
Binayak Sinha

CASE 5:	A Case of Thyrotoxic Periodic Paralysis due to Painless Thyroiditis *Debmalya Sanyal*	156
CASE 6:	Myxedema Coma: Rare but Dangerous *Soumyabrata Roy Chaudhuri*	158
CASE 7:	An Unusual Patient with Thyroiditis *Sudip Chatterjee*	162
CASE 8:	A Hyperthyroid Child *Sudip Chatterjee*	165
CASE 9:	Gynecomastia: An Unusual Initial Presentation of Thyrotoxicosis *Rana Bhattacharjee, Ajitesh Roy, Pradip Mukhopadhyay, Sujoy Ghosh*	166
CASE 10:	Two Interesting Cases of Raised Thyroid-stimulating Hormone *Sujoy Majumdar*	168

Index   171

SECTION 1

Adrenal

CASE 1: Adrenal Histoplasmosis

Tapas Chandra Das, Neeraj Sinha, Partha Sarathi Choudhury, Anirban Sinha, Animesh Maiti, Asish Kumar Basu

CASE HISTORY

A 57-year-old gentleman with diabetes mellitus for 17 years on oral antidiabetic agents, presented with complaints of weight loss (4 kg documented in 2 months), anorexia, vomiting and postural dizziness for 2 months.

Clinical examination: Conscious, oriented and afebrile; pulse rate: 78 beats/min, blood pressure: 130/80 mm Hg with significant postural drop present. Weight: 59 kg. Body mass index (BMI): 21.67 kg/m². Pigmentation present in buccal mucosa and over knuckles; rest of the systemic examination was normal.
Chest X-ray—hyperinflated lung fields; echocardiography—normal
USG abdomen + KUB: Liver, spleen—NAD, bilateral kidneys—normal, Prostate: 14 g, postvoid residual urine—insignificant

CT abdomen: Bilateral adrenal enlargement. Right side: 33 × 27 mm, left side: 42 × 24 mm. Right one enhanced by >12 HU, left one did not enhance (Fig. 1). Laboratory investigations are summarized in Table 1.

TABLE 1: Investigations.

Parameters	Value
Hemoglobin	11 g/dL
Total leukocyte count	7,300 cells/mm³
Differential leukocyte count	N60 L30 E8 M2
Platelet	3.5 lacs/mm³
Creatinine	0.8 mg/dL
Serum sodium/potassium	130/4.7 mEq/L
Fasting plasma glucose/Postprandial plasma glucose	150/283 mg/dL
Glycosylated hemoglobin	8.2%
Free thyroxine/Thyroid-stimulating hormone	1.2 ng/dL/3.2 mIU/mL
Cortisol	4.9 µg/dL
Adrenocorticotrophic hormone	191 pg/mL
Plasma renin activity	12.93 ng/mL/h (1.3–3.95 ng/mL/h)
Dehydroepiandrosterone sulfate	10.4 µg/dL (48–361 µg/dL)
Testosterone	406 ng/dL

Fine needle aspiration cytology (FNAC) adrenal: Smears show degenerated inflammatory cells and small yeast cells both intracellularly and extracellularly having the morphology of histoplasma and necrosis (histoplasmosis) (Fig. 2).

Diagnosis: A case of type 2 diabetes mellitus with adrenal histoplasmosis presenting with primary adrenal insufficiency.

In-hospital course: Patient was put on basal bolus insulin regimen and was given a 14-day course of liposomal amphotericin B followed by oral itraconazole (200 mg bd) for 1 year along with hydrocortisone replacement.

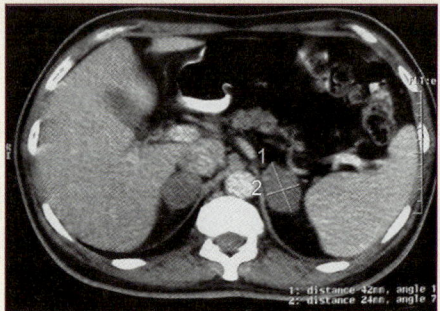
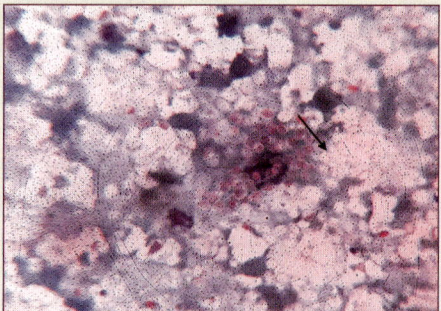

FIG. 1: Bilateral adrenal glands are enlarged. Right: 33 × 27 mm, Left: 42 × 24 mm.

FIG. 2: Smears show degenerated inflammatory cells and small yeast cells both intracellularly and extracellularly having the morphology of histoplasma and necrosis.

DISCUSSION

Weight loss in patients with diabetes is a grave concern to the clinician. It may be secondary to tuberculosis, malignancy, Graves' disease, chronic inflammatory disease, chronic diarrhea or even due to adrenal insufficiency (as in this case).

Primary adrenal insufficiency is associated with increased morbidity and mortality. Among the various causes, infective causes and autoimmune adrenalitis are more common. Worldwide infective causes are the most common causes of primary hypoadrenalism. These infective causes include tuberculosis, fungal infections (histoplasmosis, cryptococcosis), cytomegalovirus infection and human immunodeficiency virus (HIV).

Histoplasmosis is a rare (0.65% of cases) opportunistic infection in the general population and is more common in immunocompromised individuals. As diabetes mellitus is a state of immunosuppression, one should also think of histoplasmosis as a cause of primary adrenal insufficiency in these cases.

Treatment of adrenal histoplasmosis should be like that of disseminated histoplasmosis including itraconazole and amphotericin B. Glucocorticoid and mineralocorticoid replacement would be required depending upon the severity of adrenal insufficiency.

Take Home Message

- Apart from tuberculosis, malignancy and chronic inflammation, weight loss in diabetes may be due to primary adrenal insufficiency caused by opportunistic infection like histoplasmosis.

SUGGESTED READING

1. DeGroot's Text book of Endocrinology. 7th edition.
2. Harrison's Text book of Internal Medicine.19th edition. November 2014.
3. Melmed S, Polonsky KS, Larsen PR, Kronenberg HM. William's Text book of Endocrinology. 13th edition. January 2016.

CASE 2: Pheochromocytoma without Hypertension

Saurav Shishir, Chhavi Agrawal, Partha Sarathi Choudhury, Partha Pratim Chakraborty, Anirban Sinha, Animesh Maiti, Asish Kumar Basu

CASE HISTORY

A 56-year-old gentleman presented with dull-aching right upper abdominal discomfort for last 4 months. There were no associated features of weight loss, anorexia, vomiting, postural dizziness, fever, jaundice, hyperpigmentation, easy bruisability, striae, headache, palpitation, hyperhidrosis or syncope. On evaluation he was found to have a mass in the right suprarenal region on ultrasound.

Clinical examination: Pulse rate: 78 beats/min; BP: 130/80 mm Hg; no postural drop; No cushingoid stigmata; other systemic examination—Normal.

USG abdomen + KUB was suggestive of 4 × 4 cm hypoechoic SOL in right adrenal gland.

CT abdomen was suggestive of heterogeneously hyperenhancing SOL in right adrenal gland with central necrosis (Fig. 1).

Diagnosis: Normotensive pheochromocytoma

In-hospital course: Patient was started on alpha-blocker followed by beta-blocker and surgical excision of right adrenal mass was made. Intraoperative and postoperative periods were uneventful.

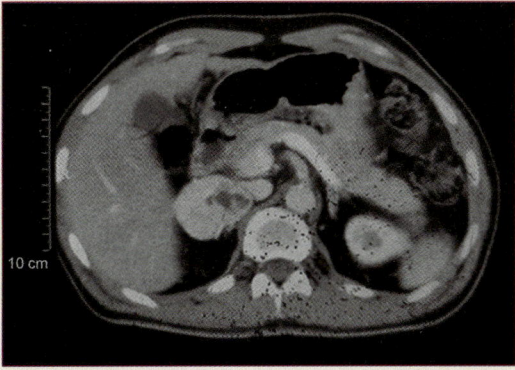

FIG. 1: CT abdomen showing heterogeneously enhancing right suprarenal SOL.

TABLE 1: Investigations.

Parametres	Value
Hemoglobin	13.3 g/dL
Total leukocyte count	6,500 cells/mm^3
Differential leukocyte count	N67 L25 E5 B1 M2
Platelets	2.5 lac/mm^3
Serum creatinine	0.8 mg/dL
Serum sodium/potassium	138/4.4 mEq/L
Total testosterone	267 ng/dL
Cortisol (overnight dexamethasone suppression test)	0.52 µg/dL
Dehydroepiandrosterone sulfate	150 µg/dL (48–361 µg/dL)
24 h urinary metanephrines	136 µg/24 h (<350)
24 h urinary nor metanephrines	4,709 µg/24 h (<600)

DISCUSSION

Sustained or paroxysmal hypertension is found in 85–90% of pheochromocytoma. Up to 13% of pheochromocytoma patients may present with persistently normal blood pressure. Proportion of normotensive pheochromocytoma is higher in patients with adrenal incidentaloma. So all patients with adrenal incidentaloma should be routinely screened for pheochromocytoma irrespective of the presence of hypertension.

Take Home Message

- As about 13% of pheochromocytoma patients are absolutely normotensive, all patients with adrenal incidentaloma should be routinely screened for pheochromocytoma.

SUGGESTED READING

1. DeGroot's Text book of Endocrinology. 7th edition.
2. Harrison's Text book of Internal Medicine. 19th edition. November 2014.
3. Nieman LK. Approach to the Patient with an Adrenal Incidentaloma. J Clin Endocrinol Metab. 2010;95(9):4106-13.
4. Melmed S, Polonsky KS, Larsen PR, Kronenberg HM. William's Text book of Endocrinology. 13th edition. January 2016.

CASE 3: A 32-year-old Man with Hypertension

JJ Mukherjee

CASE HISTORY

A 32-year-old male executive, recently married, presented to the hospital for the management of newly detected high blood pressure (BP). He had visited his general practitioner (GP) 2 weeks ago with complaints of tiredness and frequent headaches. His BP was found to be elevated at 170/110 mm Hg. His GP requested for a few investigations, and started him on amlodipine 5 mg once daily. There was no significant past medical history of note. His mother is on medications for type 2 diabetes mellitus. He does not consume tobacco in any form, and drinks alcohol only occasionally. There are no known allergies.

On examination, he was conscious, alert and oriented. There was no pallor, clubbing or icterus. His body mass index was 22.5 kg/m^2. His pulse rate was 76 beats/min, regular. His BP, checked in the right arm in a sitting position, was 164/104 mm Hg. Examination of the cardiovascular, respiratory, abdominal and central nervous system was normal.

What do you think is the likely cause of his hypertension?
The most common cause for hypertension at this age remains essential hypertension. However, in view of his age, secondary causes of hypertension need exclusion (Box 1). Among the secondary causes, obstructive sleep apnea (OSA) and renal parenchymal disease top the list. Both these conditions can be easily confirmed or excluded following clinical examination and a few basic investigations. Following this, a number of endocrine causes of hypertension need consideration. A number of these endocrine conditions causing hypertension are but obvious, such as, acromegaly, Cushing's syndrome and thyrotoxicosis, while a fair few can be easily deciphered based upon basic laboratory investigations (hypothyroidism and hyperparathyroidism). The remaining causes of endocrine hypertension call for more focused and specific investigations. Indiscriminate screening of all persons with hypertension for endocrine causes is not justified. A careful history and proper clinical examination shall point toward the situations where detailed investigations for an endocrine cause of hypertension are warranted.

Box 1: Common causes for secondary hypertension.
• Renal parenchymal disease
• Obstructive sleep apnea
• Renal artery stenosis
• Endocrine causes of hypertension (see Box 2)

What specific questions would you like to ask him and would you want to do a more detailed physical examination?
One must ask pointed questions to screen for secondary causes of hypertension. Snoring and day-time somnolence shall point toward OSA, especially in the obese individual. History of renal colic, recurrent urinary tract infections, pyuria, or hematuria can direct one to investigate for renal parenchymal disease. History of "spells", though rare, should be asked for. Past history of episodic muscle weakness or paralysis necessitating admission to a hospital should be asked. A detailed family history is mandatory.

A thorough physical examination is necessary. Feel for all peripheral pulses; absence of a few pulses is an important clue to vascular pathology. Radiofemoral delay should be specifically looked for; one might detect coarctation of aorta. Blood pressure must be measured in both arms. Look for subtle signs of acromegaly, thyrotoxicosis and Cushing's syndrome. Careful examination of the abdomen is necessary to look for any lumps, renal mass, or epigastric/flank bruit.

There was no history of snoring or daytime somnolence. There was no history of renal colic, pyuria, hematuria, or past history of recurrent urinary tract infections. There was no family history of any endocrinopathy. On examination, there was no radiofemoral delay. Blood pressure, checked in the left arm in a sitting position, was 160/100 mm Hg. There were no clinical features to suggest acromegaly, Cushing's syndrome or thyrotoxicosis. There was no abdominal bruit. The results of the investigations requested by his GP are:

Hemoglobin: 14 g/dL; serum sodium: 142 mmol/L; serum potassium: 3.8 mmol/L; serum creatinine: 0.9 mg/dL (CKD-EPI estimated glomerular filtration rate: 113 mL/min); no abnormality in routine urine examination; normal chest X-ray; no abnormality in the 12-lead-electrocardiogram (in particular, no left ventricular hypertrophy).

What further investigations would you request for next?
Following a detailed history, a thorough physical examination, and preliminary laboratory investigations, we can conclude that hypertension secondary to OSA or renal parenchymal pathology is unlikely. We need to consider endocrine causes of hypertension (Box 2). Of these, based upon clinical findings, acromegaly and Cushing's syndrome are possibly excluded. It is probably prudent to exclude thyroid and parathyroid dysfunction before proceeding to further investigations.

Serum free T4: 1.2 µg/dL (N: 0.92–1.70 µg/dL); TSH: 2.6 µIU/mL (N: 0.45–4.2 µIU/mL); serum calcium: 8.9 mg/dL (N: 8.8–104 mg/dL); serum albumin: 3.8 g/dL.

The possibilities now include mineralocorticoid-mediated hypertension (including primary hyperaldosteronism), catecholamine-secreting lesions (pheochromocytoma/paraganglioma), and renovascular hypertension.

What investigations would you request for next?
It is best to approach the possibilities step-wise, excluding one condition at-a-time. Among the three, primary hyperaldosteronism (PA) is unequivocally more common. As such, checking for plasma aldosterone concentration (PAC) and plasma renin activity (PRA) should be the next step. It would be ideal if all antihypertensive medications interfering with renin–angiotensin–aldosterone system (RAAS) could be withdrawn prior to collection of blood samples. However, in real life, it is often not possible to withdraw antihypertensive medications for fear of precipitating accelerated hypertension. As such, collect samples irrespective of the antihypertensive medications being consumed; just one caveat: mineralocorticoid receptor (MR) antagonists (spironolactone or eplerenone) must be stopped for at least 4–6 weeks prior to collecting samples for PAC and PRA.

Plasma aldosterone concentration: 12.6 ng/dL; PRA: 0.3 ng/mL/h.

At first sight, PAC is not very high, and one might overlook the possibility of PA. However, PAC must be interpreted in tandem with PRA value; one needs to calculate the aldosterone/renin ratio (ARR). It is 42 ng/dL per ng/mL/h in this case-scenario, which is highly suggestive of PA. The screening test for PA is considered positive at a certain cut-off value of ARR. The higher the ARR, the higher the chance of confirming the diagnosis of PA. While interpreting ARR, pay attention to the units in which PAC (ng/dL or pmol/L) and PRA (ng/mL/h or pmol/L/min) values are reported; also, note

> **Box 2: Endocrine causes of hypertension.**
> - Pituitary-dependent causes
>   - Cushing's disease
>   - Acromegaly
> - Thyroid-dependent causes
>   - Thyrotoxicosis (predominantly systolic hypertension)
>   - Hypothyroidism (predominantly diastolic hypertension)
> - Parathyroid-dependent causes
>   - Hyperparathyroidism
> - Adrenal-dependent causes
>   - Glucocorticoid-mediated hypertension (Cushing's syndrome)
>   - Catecholamine-mediated hypertension (pheochromocytoma/paraganglioma)
>   - Mineralocorticoid-mediated hypertension
>   - Elevated aldosterone (low renin)
>   Primary aldosteronism:
>   - Unilateral aldosterone adenoma
>   - Bilateral adrenal hyperplasia
>   - Unilateral adrenal hyperplasia
>   - Glucocorticoid remediable aldosteronism (GRA)
>   - Aldosterone-producing adrenocortical carcinoma
>   - Suppressed aldosterone (low renin)
>   Acquired:
>   - Cushing's syndrome
>   - Licorice or carbenoxolone ingestion (11-β hydroxysteroid dehydrogenase 2 inhibition)
>
>   Genetic:
>   - Syndrome of apparent mineralocorticoid excess (AME)
>   - Activating mutation of the mineralocorticoid receptor
>   - Liddle's syndrome
>   - Congenital adrenal hyperplasia (17-α hydroxylase deficiency, 11-β hydroxylase deficiency)
>   - Hyperdeoxycorticosteronism (low renin)
>   - Deoxycorticosterone producing tumor
>   - Primary cortisol resistance
>   - Congenital adrenal hyperplasia (as noted above)
>   - Elevated aldosterone (elevated renin)
>   Secondary hyperaldosteronism:
>   - Renovascular hypertension
>   - Coarctation of aorta
>   - Reninoma (very rare)

whether the laboratory has measured PRA or have they measured renin directly (direct renin concentration, DRC reported either in mU/L or ng/L). The cut-off values understandably are different depending upon the analytes being measured and the units in which they are reported.

Following a positive screening ARR, the next step concerns confirming the diagnosis of PA. One can skip this step if the ARR is unequivocally high. However, under most circumstances, a confirmatory test is a necessity. The ARR of 42 ng/dL per ng/mL/h in our case vignette is suggestive of PA but needs confirmation. The confirmatory testing strategies for PA include intravenous saline loading test, oral salt loading test, captopril challenge test and fludrocortisone suppression test. The detailed description of these tests is outside the scope of this write-up. Of these four tests, the author prefers the saline loading test.

The patient received 2 L of 0.9% saline over 4 hours, starting at 9 AM. PAC was measured after the completion of saline infusion. It was 12 ng/dL.

Post 2 L 0.9% saline infusion, PAC <5 ng/dL rules out the diagnosis of PA. PAC >10 ng/dL confirms PA; PAC between 5 ng/dL and 10 ng/dL is borderline.

Following confirmation of PA, it is essential to establish the etiology of PA to allow focused treatment. The two common differential diagnoses for PA are unilateral aldosterone-producing adenoma (APA) and bilateral idiopathic hyperaldosteronism (bilateral idiopathic hyperplasia). Rarer forms are unilateral primary adrenal hyperplasia, aldosterone-producing adrenocortical carcinomas, and familial hyperaldosteronism type 1 (glucocorticoid remediable aldosteronism). All patients with confirmed PA should have a computed tomogram (CT) of the abdomen with 3 mm cuts through the adrenal region as the initial study to establish the etiology of PA. Magnetic resonance imaging has no advantage over CT in the evaluation of the subtype of PA.

CT scan of the abdomen revealed bilateral adrenal hyperplasia (Figs. 1 and 2). In the absence of unilateral adrenal disease, surgical treatment is not an option in our case vignette. He was started on the mineralocorticoid receptor antagonist eplerenone 50 mg once daily. His blood pressure normalized at 126/80 mm Hg.

In patients with unilateral adenoma on CT, it is recommended that adrenal venous sampling (AVS) should be performed to lateralize the source of excessive aldosterone secretion prior to proceeding with surgical treatment (laparoscopic adrenalectomy). However, AVS facility is not available in most centers, is expensive, has high failure rates, and is an invasive procedure. As such, it is best to refer patients with confirmed PA (positive ARR, nonsuppression of PAC on saline suppression test) to an endocrine unit specializing in the management of endocrine hypertension to allow appropriate subtyping and directed management.

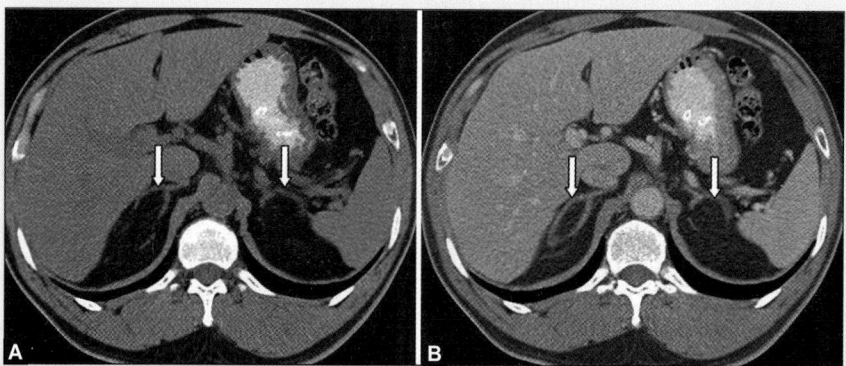

FIGS. 1A AND B: Pre- (A) and post- (B) contrast computed tomogram showing normal adrenal glands.

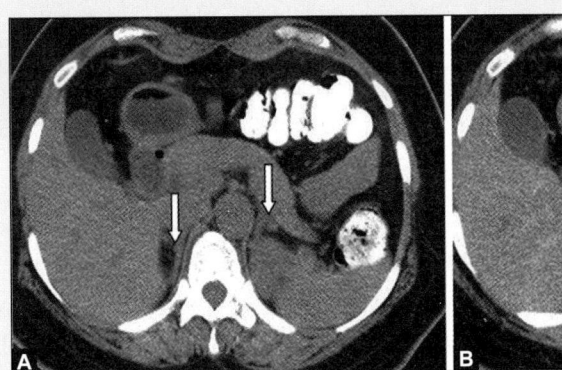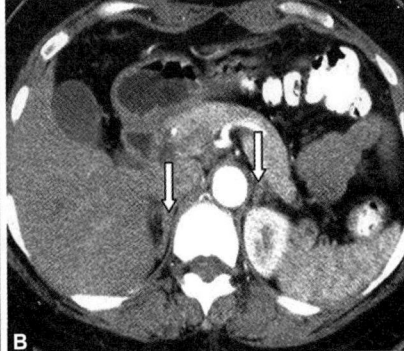

FIGS. 2A AND B: Pre- (A) and post- (B) contrast computed tomogram of the patient in discussion showing bilateral adrenal hyperplasia.

DISCUSSION

It has become increasingly clear that half to two-thirds of patients with primary aldosteronism (PA) do not present with hypokalemia. One must consider testing for PA in hypertensive patients with hypokalemia, in hypertensive patients with an adrenal incidentaloma, in diabetic patients with resistant hypertension, in young hypertensives, and in hypertensive patients who have a family history of early onset hypertension, stroke at age less than 40 years, or relatives with PA. Checking ARR, followed by a confirmatory 0.9% saline suppression test, can be undertaken at primary care level; the patient with confirmed PA could then be referred to an endocrine unit for further subtyping and treatment.

Take Home Message

- Primary aldosteronism is the most common identifiable, specifically treatable, and curable form of endocrine hypertension.

SUGGESTED READING

1. Funder JW, Carey RM, Mantero F, et al. The management of primary aldosteronism: case detection, diagnosis, and treatment: An endocrine society clinical practice guideline. J Clin Endocrinol Metab. 2016;101:1889-916.
2. Hiramatsu K, Yamada T, Yukimura Y, et al. A screening test to identify aldosterone-producing adenoma by measuring plasma renin activity. Results in hypertensive patients. Arch Intern Med. 1981;141:1589-93.
3. Mukherjee JJ, Khoo CM, Thai AC, et al. Type 2 diabetic patients with resistant hypertension should be screened for primary aldosteronism. Diab Vasc Dis Res 2010;7:6-13.
4. Stowasser M, Gordon RD. The aldosterone-renin ratio for screening for primary aldosteronism. Endocrinologist. 2004;14:267-76.
5. Young WF, Calhoun DA, Lenders JWM, et al. Screening for endocrine hypertension: an endocrine society scientific statement. Endocrine Reviews. 2017;38:103-22.

CASE 4

Giddiness and Near-syncope Post Pacemaker Implantation—Not Always Cardiac or Neurogenic

Soumyabrata Roy Chaudhuri

CASE HISTORY

A 70-year-old muslim lady suffering from hypothyroid, already on levothyroxine supplement, was admitted to the ICU of a charitable trust run hospital in August 2018 with complaints of intermittent syncope. She was seen to have complete heart block on the ECG and was promptly taken to the catheter laboratory and a temporary pulse generator was inserted via the transfemoral route after hyperkalemia was excluded (potassium value read 4.6 mEq/L via the arterial blood gas machine also equipped to deliver electrolyte reports). She was discharged 3 days after permanent pacemaker implantation as per protocol by the Consultant In-charge and was asked to follow-up in OPD.

She was readmitted in the ICU of the same institute again in early January 2019, with extreme weakness, nausea and occasional vomiting, abdominal pain, loss of weight and multiple episodes of giddiness and one episode of faintness. In the meanwhile she was seen by her primary care physician who had put her onto levetiracetam 500 mg thrice daily to guard against absence seizures but she did not show any symptomatic improvement. TSH was checked and the value being 6.62 U/dL, levothyroxine supplementation was increased to 75 μg/day.

Ultrasonography of the abdomen was unremarkable except for mild hepatomegaly with fatty infiltration of liver and cortical cyst right kidney and the chest X-ray was noncontributory. The pulse generator was thoroughly checked for any dysfunction or exit block but nothing was revealed. Baseline investigations were normal except for the creatinine, sodium and potassium (Table 1). For evaluating the hyponatremia—Free T4, TSH and at 8 AM cortisol was sent. Free T4 was 1.24 u/dL, TSH was 3.2 u/dL whereas 8 AM cortisol was 4.91 μg/dL. Urinary spot sodium was 86. She was started on hydrocortisone 100 mg intravenous after blood for ACTH was sent and an anti-TPO antibody was also sent along with. There was dramatic improvement of symptoms within 24 hours.

After 48 hours she was started on hydrocortisone tablets 10 mg in the morning and 5 mg each in the afternoon and night. Hydration had already brought her creatinine down to 1.0 mg/dL and urea to 42 mg/dL, blood pressure was stable at 120–130 mm Hg systolic and 70–75 mm Hg diastolic and a contrast-enhanced CT scan of the abdomen was done which showed hepatosplenomegaly, diffuse fatty changes in the liver, normal sized adrenals without any focal lesion. The patient made drastic recovery with hydrocortisone and by day 5 patient was up and about with serum sodium at 127 mEq/L and potassium at 4.6 mEq/L. ACTH values came in the normal range 22.94 pg/mL (morning range 7.2–63.3 pg/mL) thereby indicating that this was a case of secondary hypocortisolemia (since there was no rise of ACTH in response to the low levels of cortisol). Anti-TPO antibody was positive.

As the pulse generator was of a basic nature without MRI compatibility, MRI of the pituitary could not be done. Keeping the financial constraints in mind the patient was

Section 1: Adrenal

TABLE 1: Investigation reports.

Test	Report	Normal range
Urea	98 mg/dL	(7–20)
Serum creatinine	1.9 mg/dL	(0.7–1.2)
Serum sodium	115 mEq/L	(137–148)
Serum potassium	5.1 mEq/L	(3.5–5.0)
Bilirubin	0.6 mg/dL	(up to 1.2)
Serum glutamic-pyruvic transaminase	14 U/L	(<41)
Serum glutamic-oxaloacetic transaminase	17 U/L	(<37)
Total protein	7.8 g/dL	(6.6–8.3)
Albumin	3.9 g/dL	(3.5–5.5)
Globulin	3.1 g/dL	(2–3.5)
Serum amylase	62 U/L	(22–80)
Serum lipase	112 U/L	(<67 U/L)
Hemoglobin	11.2 g/L	(13–17)
Total leukocyte count	7,800 cells/mm^3	(4.5–11.0)
Neutrophil	65%	(40–80)
Blood pressure	90/70 mm Hg	

released with the advice of checking the other pituitary hormones (FSH, LH, prolactin and IGF1), and doing a CT scan of the pituitary fossa. The patient had visited the pacemaker follow-up clinic but is yet to turn up with the hormonal profile and CT scan results.

DISCUSSION

Addison's disease is a relatively rare condition with an annual incidence of 4 million in the western population and is difficult to diagnose due to the presentation with nonspecific symptoms. The wide variety of symptoms means that the diagnosis may be attributed to numerous other conditions as the more cardinal symptoms like skin or mucous membrane pigmentation may be missed or may not be present at all.

A clinician may suspect the diagnosis and send for a random cortisol estimation which however may be inaccurate due to the circadian rhythm of cortisol production. An unusually low cortisol in the presence of clinical features of Addison's disease should raise a suspicion about the diagnosis and this may be confirmed by a trial of hydrocortisone, however cortisol and ACTH should be sent for before the administration of steroids (Tables 2 and 3). Raised TSH may be a feature and sometimes Addison's disease may be worsened by starting or increasing dose of thyroxine. Routine blood may show hyponatremia, and/or hypokalemia, hypoglycemia and eosinophilia. Anorexia or hypotension may be relevant but are nonspecific.

TABLE 2: When to think Addison's.

Key diagnostic factors	Other diagnostic factors	Risk factors
Presence of risk factors	Nausea	Female sex
Fatigue	Vomiting	Adrenocortical autoantibodies
Anorexia	Hypotension	Adrenal hemorrhage
Weight loss	Arthralgia and myalgia	Autoimmune diseases

TABLE 3: Investigations to confirm diagnosis.

First investigations to order	Investigations to consider
Serum electrolytes	Adrenocorticotrophic hormone (ACTH) stimulation test
Blood urea	Serum ACTH
Complete blood count	Plasma renin activity
Morning serum cortisol	Plasma aldosterone

Autoimmune polyendocrine syndrome (APS) refers to multiple endocrine gland insufficiency associated with autoimmune disease. It is, however, also used to describe syndromes characterized by the association of two or more organ specific disorders. Genetic inheritance such as autoimmune regulator (AIRE) gene in APS type 1 or polygenic inheritance in APS type II has also come up in recent times.

Autoimmune polyendocrine syndrome type 1 is an autosomal recessive disorder and is characterized by the association of Addison's disease, hypoparathyroidism and chronic candidiasis; however, other associations like vitiligo, hepatitis, pernicious anemia, atrophic gastritis and type 1 diabetes mellitus (T1DM) are also seen. APS type II (aka Schmidt's syndrome) is more common than the type I variant and is associated with conditions including Addison's disease, T1DM and autoimmune thyroid disease. It is associated with HLA-DR3 and DR4.

Take Home Message

- *Despite pacemaker insertion if giddiness presyncope or fall occurs please think addison's in addition to ruling out neurogenic or neurocardiogenic syncope.*

SUGGESTED READING

1. Puttanna A, Cunningham AR, Dainty P, et al. Addison's disease and its associations. BMJ Case Rep. 2013;2013:bcr2013010473.

CASE 5: Triple A Syndrome

Rana Bhattacharjee, Pradip Mukhopadhyay, Sujoy Ghosh

CASE HISTORY

An 11-year-old girl presented with history of intermittent vomiting, generalized weakness and increased skin pigmentation over the last 2 years. She was born of nonconsanguineous marriage. She was delivered vaginally with breech presentation. There was no adverse perinatal event. Developmental milestones were normal. There was no family history of similar illness.

Six months prior to this presentation she was admitted to a hospital with recurrent vomiting and diarrhea. She was diagnosed to have primary adrenal insufficiency and started on hydrocortisone tablets and referred to IPGMER, Kolkata for further evaluation.

On further enquiry, the parents said that they had noticed reduced production of tears since early childhood. Over the last few weeks she was also experiencing difficulty in swallowing both solids and liquids.

On examination, she was thinly built and had hyperpigmentation of the skin and mucous membranes. Her height was 126.3 cm (<3rd centile). Mid-parental target height was 149.7 cm (25th to 50th centile). Her blood pressure was 74/66 mm Hg on supine position and 70/58 mm Hg on standing position. Her breast and pubic hair were prepubertal. There were no axillary hairs. She had photophobia. Lacrimal gland was not visible on clinical examination (Fig. 1). Schirmer's test was positive [4 mm (N >10 mm)]. Other systemic examination was unremarkable.

Investigations revealed hemoglobin 11.5 g/dL, TLC: 8,300 cells/mm^3, polymorphs: 46%, lymphocyte: 49%, eosinophil: 5%. Fasting plasma glucose: 91 mg/dL, sodium: 136 mEq/L, potassium: 3.9 mEq/L, urea: 20 mg/dL, creatinine: 0.3 mg/dL, normal liver function tests, ACTH: 1,115 pg/mL, morning cortisol <1 µg/dL. TSH: 8.9 mIU/L, Free T4: 1.1 ng/dL. Plasma renin activity: 2.8 (0.29–4.1 ng/mL/h).

Barium swallow X-ray esophagus was suggestive of achalasia cardia (Fig. 2) which was subsequently confirmed by esophageal manometry studies.

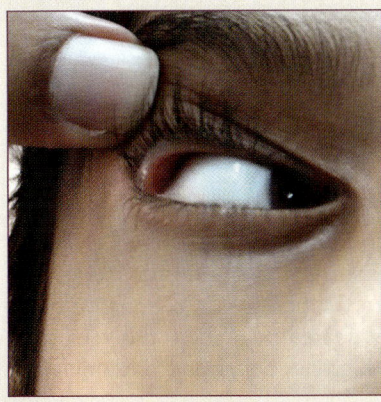

FIG. 1: Absent lacrimal gland (alacrima).

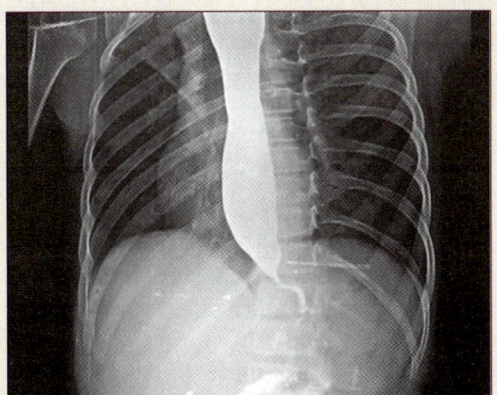

FIG. 2: Achalasia cardia demonstrated by barium swallow X-ray.

INTRODUCTION

Allgrove's syndrome or Triple A syndrome was first described by Allgrove and colleagues in 1978 in two pairs of unrelated siblings and is characterized by achalasia, alacrima and adrenocorticotropic hormone (ACTH)-resistant adrenal failure. Other associated features can be autonomic nervous system abnormalities, short stature, glossitis, angular cheilitis, fissured tongue and microcephaly. The syndrome is associated with mutations in the *AAAS* gene located on chromosome 12 q13 whose product is ALADIN (alacrima-achalasia-adrenal insufficiency-neurologic disorder). Clinical presentation can be widely variable.

DISCUSSION

Primary adrenal insufficiency is not very common in children. Triple A syndrome or Allgrove's syndrome is a very rare cause of primary adrenocortical insufficiency in children. It is characterized by a combination of achalasia, alacrima and ACTH resistance. Mineralocorticoid secretion is usually normal because it is regulated by RAAS rather than hypothalamo–pituitary–adrenal axis. The index patient presented with classical triad of Allgrove's syndrome along with short stature. Early recognition of this syndrome leads to effective management of the condition.

Take Home Messages

- *Primary adrenocortical insufficiency is a rare disorder in children*
- *Triple A or Allgrove's syndrome is manifested by resistance to ACTH, alacrima, and achalasia along with variable presence of other organ involvement*
- *Thorough search for these associated clinical clues should be undertaken when a child present with primary adrenocortical insufficiency (particularly in those with sparing of mineralocorticoid axis).*

CASE 6: Evolving Primary Adrenal Insufficiency*

Rana Bhattacharjee, Ajitesh Roy, Pradip Mukhopadhyay, Sujoy Ghosh

CASE HISTORY

A 31-year-old male presented with fever and weight loss for 3.5 months with loss of appetite, nausea, progressive darkening of skin and profound generalized weakness without any history of chronic cough or hemoptysis. There was no history suggestive of any autoimmune endocrine disease or any history suggestive of connective tissue diseases or vasculitis. A past history of adequately treated pulmonary tuberculosis at the age of 3 years was present. There is no history high-risk behavior. On examination,

---

*With permission from: Roy A, Bhattacharjee R, Ghosh S, et al. Evolving adrenal insufficiency. Indian J Endocrinol Metab. 2012;16(Suppl 2):S369-70.

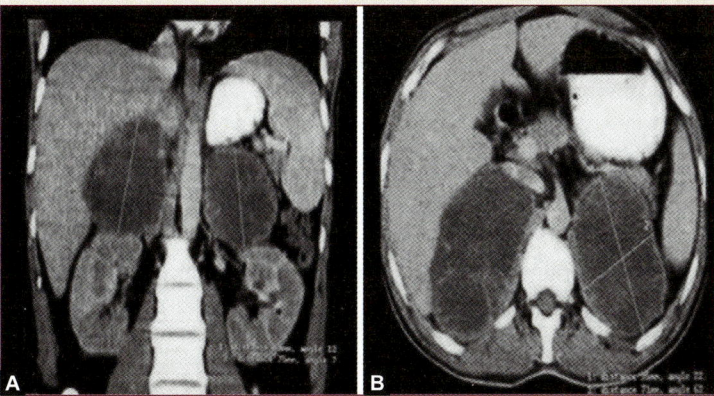

FIGS. 1A AND B: CT scan of the abdomen (coronal and axial).

patient was anemic with stable vitals without any postural drop of blood pressure. A nontender, firm lymph node over the right submandibular region was found. There was hyperpigmentation of the skin and buccal mucosa. The patient was febrile but systemic survey was unremarkable (Fig. 1).

Investigations: Hemoglobin (Hb): 10.4 g/dL, erythrocyte sedimentation rate (ESR): 70 mm/h, fasting blood sugar (FBS): 86 mg/dL with normal renal function and electrolytes. Liver function test (LFT) was normal except increased alkaline phosphate (495 U/L), X-ray chest: Normal.

HIV: Negative, sputum for AFB: Negative.

On day 10 (D10) after admission:
Cortisol (8 AM) = 19.9 µg/dL, ACTH: 197.1 pg/mL

On day 22 after admission:
Cortisol (8 AM): 7.9 µg/dL. Cortisol after 30 minutes of injection tetracosactrin (synacthen): 10.5 µg/dL.

Thyroid function test: Within normal limits; CT scan of abdomen: Bilateral heterogenous hypodense adrenal mass (Right: 10.68 × 7.6 × 8.8 cm; Left: 9.5 × 7.1 × 7.5 cm).

CT-guided FNAC from adrenals: Inconclusive. Stain and culture for AFB and histoplasma were negative. FNAC from enlarged cervical lymph node revealed caseating granuloma without any demonstrable AFB.

The patient was provisionally diagnosed as evolving primary adrenal insufficiency (due to possible tubercular etiology) after initial paired cortisol and ACTH report which showed cortisol level of >18.5 µg/dL in the face of high ACTH level. Differential diagnosis of histoplasmosis and adrenal metastasis were considered, but ruled out by negative fungal culture and stain, and negative history of primary malignancy and noncontributory FNA.

The lymphadenopathy regressed and general well-being improved with a decrease in skin pigmentation following treatment with ATDs and appropriate glucocorticoid and fludrocortisone replacement. After 1 year of treatment, steroid withdrawal was attempted,

> but was not successful and adrenal size was almost the same as last CT scan (Right: 9.7 × 9.2 cm; Left: 10.4 × 8 cm). Even after 2 years of follow-up, the adrenal size did not regress and he was on/continued glucocorticoid and mineralocorticoid supplementation.

INTRODUCTION

Tuberculosis is one of the most common causes of Addison's disease. Adrenal reserve in tuberculosis is still an enigma and recovery of adrenal function is unpredictable.

DISCUSSION

Tuberculosis is known to affect adrenal glands directly to cause Addison's disease. Rich vascularity and the high levels of local corticosteroids that suppress cell-mediated immunity (CMI) make the adrenal gland an ideal nidus for *Mycobacterium tuberculosis*. Adrenal tuberculosis is seen in up to 6% of patients with active tuberculosis and is usually bilateral. Adrenal destruction by tuberculosis may lead to overt or subclinical adrenal insufficiency and it may present in an evolving state which was observed in this case. The adrenal cortex has considerable capacity to regenerate with marked hyperplasia and hypertrophy of cortical cells, noted during the period of active infection. Ultimately fibrosis ensues and the adrenals become normal or smaller in size with calcification evident in 50% of cases after the disease becomes inactive.

In cases of tubercular adrenalitis, CT scans of the abdomen shows typical features of shrunken and calcified adrenals in chronic stage and enlargement in the active stage. However, in the present case, they failed to regress.

Reversal of adrenal function following antitubercular therapy is a controversial issue. While some of the studies have shown normalization of adrenal function following therapy in a large number of cases, other studies have contradicted it. If the adrenal size remains the same (as it is in this case), it is prudent to follow the patient up for recovery of adrenal function and size.

CONCLUSION

Evolving adrenal insufficiency is suspected when a patient present with clinical features of primary adrenal insufficiency, high ACTH with apparently normal cortisol level. Such patients have high risk of progression to overt adrenocortical insufficiency. The adrenal has considerable capacity to regenerate during active infection and ultimately become normal or smaller in size. However, in the case reported here, they failed to regress over 2 years. Reversal of adrenal function following ATD is controversial.

> **Take Home Messages**
> - *In a patient with suspected primary adrenocortical insufficiency, high ACTH with apparently normal cortisol level suggest evolving adrenocortical insufficiency*
> - *Such patients need close follow-up for early detection of overt adrenocortical insufficiency*
> - *In many of the patients of tubercular adrenalitis, even after completion of course of antitubarcular drugs, adrenal function may not recover.*

SECTION 2
Bones

CASE 1: Pseudofracture (Looser's Zone) with Subsequent Low Trauma Fracture: Under-recognized but not Uncommon Presentation of Distal Renal Tubular Acidosis

Subhankar Chowdhury, Partha Pratim Chakraborty

CASE HISTORY

In recent past two postmenopausal ladies in their early 50s were referred for preoperative evaluation before open reduction and internal fixation of subtrochanteric femur fractures. Baseline investigations including albumin corrected serum calcium, phosphorus and vitamin D concentrations were normal. Plain radiographs revealed bilateral Looser's zone in both of them that had been overlooked previously in the first lady (Fig. 1). The radiograph in the second lady also demonstrated right-sided nephrocalcinosis (Fig. 2). A detailed history documented that they had been suffering from myalgia, some amount of proximal muscle weakness and generalized aches

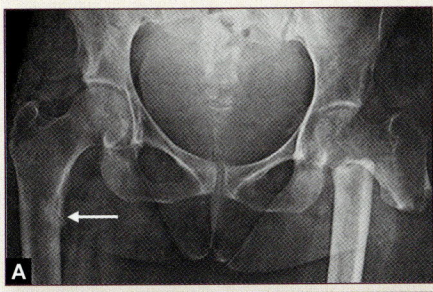
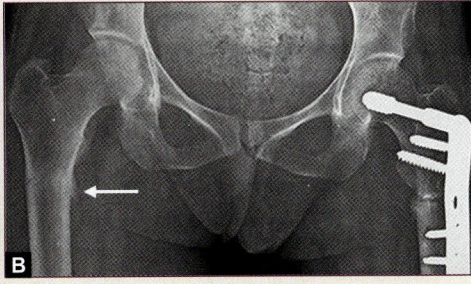
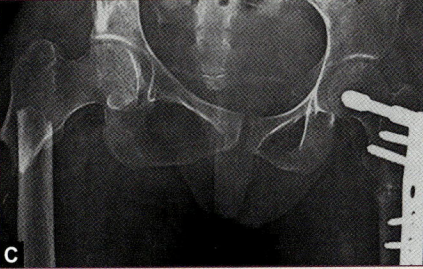

FIGS. 1A TO C: Initial radiograph of the first lady showing left-sided subtrochanteric fracture (panel A) that had been managed with open reduction and internal fixation (panel B). Looser's zone over the right femur had been overlooked since her first presentation (arrows in panels A and B) that ultimately resulted in right-sided subtrochanteric fracture (panel C).

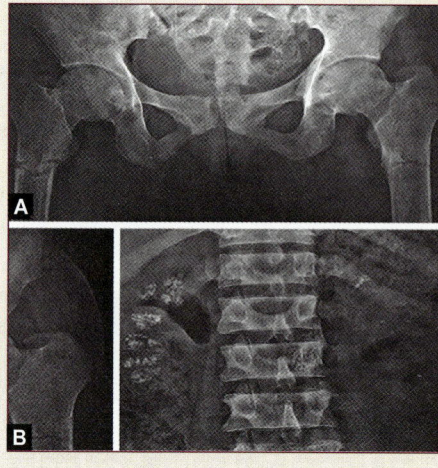
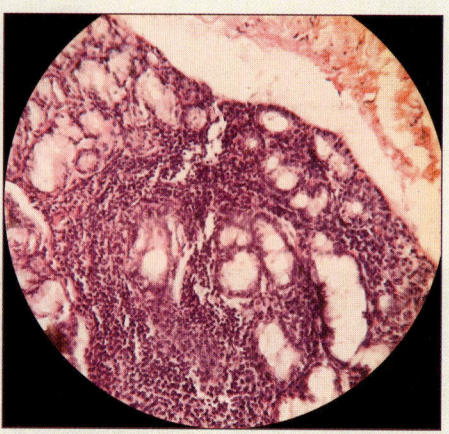

FIGS. 2A AND B: Radiograph of the second lady with subtrochanteric fracture on the right and Looser's zone on the left femur (panel A). Right-sided nephrocalcinosis is also evident in straight X-ray abdomen with probable nephrocalcinosis on the left side as well.

FIG. 3: Lymphocytic infiltration of minor salivary glands in one of the lip biopsy specimens.

TABLE 1: Summary of relevant investigations.

Parameters (Normal range)	Case 1	Case 2
Serum potassium (mmol/L) (3.5–5.5)	3.1	2.9
Arterial pH (7.35–7.45)	7.26	7.28
Anion gap (12 ± 4)	12	14
Serum bicarbonate (mmol/L) (22–26)	14	17
Urine pH	6	6.3
Urine anion gap	Positive	Positive
Ultrasonography of abdomen	Bilateral nephrocalcinosis	Bilateral nephrocalcinosis
Antinuclear antibody	Negative	Negative
Anti-SSa (anti-Ro) antibody	Positive	Positive
Anti-SSb (anti-La) antibody	Positive	Positive

and pains since long followed by low trauma fractures. They also revealed irritation of their eyes and oral cavities which had been ignored by them. Relevant investigations performed subsequently are summarized in Table 1.

Schirmer's test confirmed the presence of dry eyes and inner lip biopsy showed lymphocytic infiltration of the minor salivary glands (Fig. 3) in both of them.

DISCUSSION

Renal tubular acidosis (RTA), characterized by hyperchloremic normal anion gap metabolic acidosis, is of two types: type 1 or distal and type 2 or proximal. Both the forms can be primary or secondary to other systemic diseases and their presentations can be varied and multisystemic.

Distal RTA (dRTA) is characterized by impaired distal tubular acid secretion due to decreased activity of the H^+-ATPase pump leading to an inability to excrete the daily acid load, resulting in progressive H^+ retention and consequent metabolic acidosis. The diagnosis of dRTA is made by the simultaneous presence of alkaline urine (urine pH >5.5) in association with systemic acidosis. Hypokalemia, nephrocalcinosis, nephrolithiasis and growth failure are the common manifestations of dRTA; however, monosymptomatic presentation is not uncommon and thus poses a diagnostic challenge. Bones can also be involved secondary to chronic metabolic acidosis. Primary Sjögren's syndrome is an autoimmune disease involving predominantly the lacrimal and the salivary glands and about two-thirds of patients develop extraglandular manifestations. Clinically significant renal involvement is seen about 5% cases and tubular disorders like interstitial nephritis and dRTA predominate. Cases of proximal tubular dysfunction with/without Fanconi's syndrome, type 2 RTA and glomerular disease have also been reported. Osteomalacia, a form of metabolic bone disease, is characterized by inadequate mineralization of the bone matrix and subsequent softening of bones. The leading causes of osteomalacia are abnormal vitamin D, calcium and phosphate homeostasis secondary to nutritional deficiency or a variety of intestinal and renal disorders. Metabolic acidosis itself can give rise to osteomalacia at times by altering the local milieu and interfering with mineralization of the osteoids. Previous retrospective series from this part of the world have shown that RTA secondary to Sjögren's syndrome is often diagnosed late in spite of suggestive clues in a vast majority of them.

The most common presentations of osteomalacia are muscle weakness and ache and pains, which are often vague and thus make the correct diagnosis difficult. Looser's zone or pseudofracture, seen on plain radiography, is an important clue to the underlying osteomalacia and early diagnosis forestalls future fracture.

Take Home Messages

- *Pseudofracture is an important radiological clue to osteomalacia and such patients having normal albumin corrected calcium, phosphorus and vitamin D should be evaluated for underlying metabolic acidosis*
- *A vigorous and systemic search for primary etiology is warranted for all individuals with adult onset distal renal tubular acidosis; Sjögren's syndrome should be ruled out in all such patients*
- *Early diagnosis of metabolic acidosis as the underlying cause of osteomalacia is of utmost importance as appropriate management is quite cheap and very much effective in avoiding the dreaded complications of femur fractures, particularly in elderly individuals.*

SUGGESTED READING

1. Goules AV, Tatouli IP, Moutsopoulos HM, et al. Clinically significant renal involvement in primary Sjögren's syndrome: clinical presentation and outcome. Arthritis Rheum. 2013;65:2945-53.
2. Ramos-Casals M, Solans R, Rosas J, et al. Primary Sjögren syndrome in Spain: clinical and immunologic expression in 1010 patients. Medicine (Baltimore). 2008;87:210-9.
3. Sandhya P, Danda D, Rajaratnam S, Thomas N. Sjögren's, Renal Tubular Acidosis And Osteomalacia - An Asian Indian Series. Open Rheumatol J. 2014;8:103-9.

CASE 2: Refractory Rickets due to Fanconi's Syndrome Secondary to Wilson's Disease*

Chitra Selvan, Rana Bhattacharjee, Pradip Mukhopadhyay, Sujoy Ghosh

CASE HISTORY

A 13-year-old girl, first in birth order, born of a nonconsanguineous marriage with normal perinatal history and developmental milestones, presented with complaints of an insidious onset of progressive weakness involving both lower limbs in the form of a difficulty in getting up from a squatting position for last 6 years. She also noticed pain in her hips and lower limbs with a gradual development of knock-knees over the same period. She had pain and discomfort in her elbow and knee joints also. Her dietary intake included about 450 mL of milk per day. Sun exposure was adequate. She had received multiple doses of vitamin D sachets over past 6 years with minimal improvement. There was no history of tingling around the mouth or fingertips. She denied any history of polyuria, swelling of lower limbs, jaundice, persistent diarrhea, or intake of any relevant drugs. There was also no history of similar complaints among the other family members. Examination revealed an oriented, alert, poorly built, poorly nourished child (weight: 18.6 kg, <3rd percentile) with severe short stature (height: 120 cm <3rd percentile, SDS: −5.43, target height: 146 cm, SDS: −2.48), mildly pale, nonicteric and stable vitals. Examination of musculoskeletal system revealed widening and tenderness of wrists with valgus deformity at knees (Fig. 1). Examination of the central nervous system revealed normal mental functions, normal cranial nerves and sensory system. Examination of the motor system showed normal tone and decreased power (4/5) in the muscle groups in all limbs with normal reflexes. The patient also had a palpable liver with a span of 11 cm without any nodularity or tenderness. No palpable spleen or shifting dullness was noted. Biochemical evaluation revealed mild microcytic hypochromic anemia, normal renal functions, normal transaminases, low albumin, hypokalemia, elevated bone-specific alkaline phosphatase, normal albumin adjusted calcium, hypophosphatemia, and adequate levels of 25-hydroxyvitamin D (Table 1). Twenty-four-hour urine levels of phosphate and creatinine were 290 mg and 277 mg respectively. Tubular maximum reabsorption of phosphate per unit of glomerular filtrate (TmP/GFR) was low at 1.4 mg/dL, indicating a renal loss of phosphate. Arterial blood gas analysis revealed normal anion gap metabolic acidosis with a urine pH of 7. Skeletal radiography revealed epiphyseal dysgenesis with a loss of horizontal trabeculations at both the femoral necks, pseudofractures around the knees, and widening of epiphysis of both knees and wrists (Fig. 2).

She was found to have glucosuria in the presence of normal blood sugars and aminoaciduria, thus suggesting a diagnosis of Fanconi's syndrome. Ammonium chloride challenge test showed adequate urinary acidification, suggesting the dysfunction at proximal tubule. To screen for causes of Fanconi's syndrome, a slit-lamp examination was done and it revealed the presence of Kayser-Fleischer rings which prompted an evaluation

---

*With permission from: Chitra S, Bhattacharjee R, Ghosh S, et al. Refractory rickets due to Fanconi's Syndrome secondary to Wilson's disease. Indian J Endocrinol Metab. 2012;16(Suppl 2):S399-401.

for Wilson's disease (Fig. 3). Serum ceruloplasmin levels were low and 24-hour urine copper levels were high (Table 1). A detailed examination of the central nervous system revealed spastic dysarthria. Ultrasonography of the abdomen showed a normal-sized liver with coarse architecture, portal vein, spleen and kidneys were normal. Prothrombin time and upper gastrointestinal endoscopy were normal. Magnetic resonance (MR) imaging of the brain showed bilateral symmetrical hyperintensities in T2-weighted images in the basal ganglia, midbrain, periaqueductal areas, cerebellum and the frontal lobes consistent with Wilson's disease. Thus, a diagnosis of short stature and refractory rickets due to Fanconi's syndrome secondary to Wilson's disease was made.

She was started on a replacement of potassium and alkali in the form of potassium Shohl's solution 20 mL thrice a day and replacement of phosphate with Joulie's solution. Wilson's disease was treated with zinc acetate tablets 50 mg three times a day.

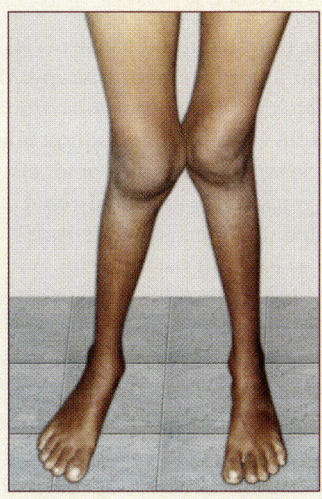

FIG. 1: Genu valgum deformity.

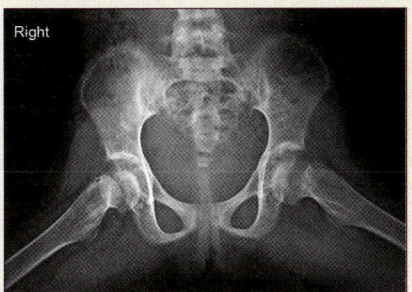

FIG. 2: X-ray of hip joint showing femoral epiphyseal dysgenesis and loss of horizontal trabeculations suggestive of rickets.

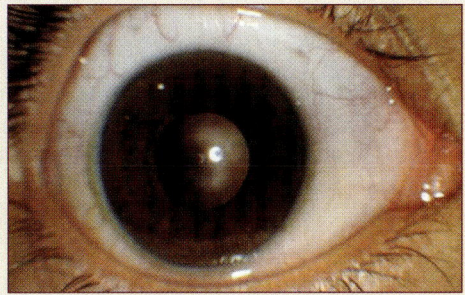

FIG. 3: Kayser-Fleischer ring.

TABLE 1: Investigations.

Tests	Value
Corrected calcium	9.24 mg/dL
Serum phosphate	2.76 mg/dL
Alkaline phosphatase	1,245 U/L, >80% bone origin
25-hydroxyvitamin D	57.2 ng/dL
Serum creatinine	0.55 mg/dL
Serum potassium	2.72 mEq/L
Urine routine examination	pH 7, sugar and amino acid present
Serum ceruloplasmin	6.5 mg/dL (18–35 mg/dL)
24-h urine phosphate	290 mg
24-h urine creatinine	277 mg
24-h urine copper	433 µg (<50 µg/24 h)

INTRODUCTION

The most common cause of rickets in children is deficiency of vitamin D and it responds well to replacement therapy. When clinical features and biochemical findings do not match for a diagnosis of vitamin D deficiency rickets, replacement of vitamin D is ineffective. In such situation a detailed search for other etiologies like hypophosphatemic rickets, renal tubular acidosis, renal osteodystrophy, and vitamin D-resistant rickets is warranted. Proximal renal tubular acidosis when accompanied by other proximal tubular defects like glucosuria, aminoaciduria, uricosuria and phosphaturia is referred to as Fanconi's syndrome.

It is a rare but important cause of short stature and hypophosphatemic rickets. Fanconi's syndrome can either be a primary abnormality in the proximal renal tubular cells or secondary to other disorders in which toxic metabolic substances lead to the derangement of tubular functions, e.g. cystinosis, Wilson's disease, tyrosinemia, galactosemia, and Lowe's syndrome. Wilson's disease is an inherited disease involving a defect of copper transport by the hepatic lysosomes which leads to excess deposition of copper in the organs, with hepatic and neuropsychiatric manifestations being the presenting feature. Rickets as the presenting feature of Wilson's disease has been reported very rarely.

We present here a child with refractory rickets due to Fanconi's syndrome secondary to Wilson's disease.

DISCUSSION

Though the majority of rickets is due to deficiency of vitamin D, it is important to be vigilant of the cases where clinical feature and biochemical findings do not corroborate with the diagnosis. In a review of refractory rickets in nonazotemic Indian patients, renal tubular diseases accounted for about a third of the cases. Rickets and osteomalacia are more common in Fanconi's syndrome as compared to other renal tubular diseases. Though exact prevalence of Wilson's disease is not known in our country, it is believed to be underreported and may have a different clinical profile in terms of presentations in the first or second decade, and the musculoskeletal form is more common. Making an etiological diagnosis of Wilson's disease is important because it is one of the few conditions which, on treatment, may lead to improvement of tubular function over time.

Take Home Messages

- Although vitamin D deficiency is a common cause of rickets, one should investigate for refractory rickets when serum vitamin D level is normal or patient doesn't improve with usual vitamin D replacement therapy
- Fanconi's syndrome can cause rickets by multiple mechanisms including phosphaturia and acidosis
- Underlying cause of proximal tubular dysfunction should be sought.

SECTION 3
Development

CASE 1: A Short Girl with Delayed Puberty
Anirban Mazumdar

CASE HISTORY

A 16-year-old girl of short stature was presented with recently detected diabetes in endocrine clinic. She was a known case of hemoglobin E-beta thalassemia (HbE/β-thalassemia) since the age of 18 months and was maintained on monthly blood transfusions since that age. Her sister and mother were carriers of E heterozygous and father was carrier of β thalassemia. She was on hydroxyurea along with deferasirox, folic acid and calcium supplementation with poor compliance because of cost. Splenectomy was performed when she was 5 years old as the requirement of transfusions increased suddenly. Nine months following her splenectomy, she became stable with monthly transfusions again. She was short since her childhood, but the family was never interested in her height as they were much preoccupied with her treatment for thalassemia. She had not attained menarche at the time of presentation. She had no family history of diabetes.

She was 141.5 cm in height (SD score −2.5 cm), 32 kg in weight, with regular and normal pulse and blood pressure. Her mid-parental height was 152 cm. She had a thalassemic facies with frontal bossing, prominent facial bones, depressed nasal bridge, mild facial puffiness accompanied by pallor. She had no icterus, and chest and cardiovascular system examination was normal. She had no pubertal development. Her breasts were of Tanner stage 1 with absent pubic and axillary hair. The following evaluations were done at the time of presentation (Table 1).

TABLE 1: Laboratory parameters.

Investigations	Results	Normal range
Hemoglobin	9.8 g/dL	12–16
Total leukocyte count	11,700 mm^3	3,500–11,000
Erythrocyte sedimentation rate	43 mm/h in women	0–29
Serum ferritin	5612.13 ng/mL	12–150
Fasting plasma glucose	312 mg/dL	70–99
Postprandial plasma glucose	495 mg/dL	70–139
Glycosylated hemoglobin	11%	3.6–5.6
Serum glutamic-pyruvic transaminase	43.2 U/L	0–38
Serum glutamic-oxaloacetic transaminase	38.4 U/L	0–31

TABLE 2: Laboratory parameters on follow-up.

Tests	Value	Normal range
Fasting plasma glucose	126 mg/dL	70–99
C-peptide (fasting)	0.5 mEq/L	135–145
C-peptide (post meal)	0.6 mEq/L	3.5–5
Anti-GAD antibody	-ve	–
Anti-IA-A2 antibody	-ve	–
Free thyroxine	1.16 ng/dL	0.9–1.6
Thyroid-stimulating hormone	2.1 µU/mL	0.4–4.8
Estradiol	16.23 pg/mL	30–160
Follicle-stimulating hormone	3.2 IU/L	1–11
Luteinizing hormone	2.1 IU/L	3–20
Cortisol (9 AM)	11.2 µg/dL	5–25
Pelvic ultrasonography	Uterus prepubertal with 3.2 cm in length and 1.3 cm in width/ovaries undetectable	

(Anti-GAD: anti-glutamic acid decarboxylase; Anti-IA-A2: islet tyrosine phosphatase 2 antibodies)

Basal-bolus insulin therapy was started for glycemic control with weekly monitoring of blood sugar and readjustment of doses. Within 1 month, her glycemic status fairly improved when she was evaluated for pancreatic β-cell functional reserve with fasting and post meal C-peptide, β-cell autoantibodies along with other hormonal profiles (Table 2).

In view of poor C-peptide response, her basal-bolus insulin therapy was continued and was monitored by weekly 4 point capillary blood glucose measurement. Her glycemic status was fairly controlled without any episode of hyperglycemic crisis. Monthly blood transfusions along with iron chelation therapy were also continued to maintain her hemoglobin and control her ferritin level respectively. Hormonal profile was suggestive of hypogonadotropic ovarian failure. But her thyroid function and serum cortisol tests were normal. She was not evaluated for growth hormone. Estrogen replacement therapy was started for low estradiol level to induce pubertal changes.

After 3 years of therapy, her serum ferritin came down to 658 ng/mL, hemoglobin was maintained at 8.4 g/dL, height increased to 145.5 cm, and body weight to 40.3 kg. Estrogen replacement therapy increased her breast size to Tanner stage 3 (Fig. 1) but without any pubic (Tanner stage 1) or axillary hair growth. She did not experience any breakthrough bleeding with estrogen therapy in 3 years. Progesterone was added after 3 years of estrogen therapy to induce regular cycle bleeding.

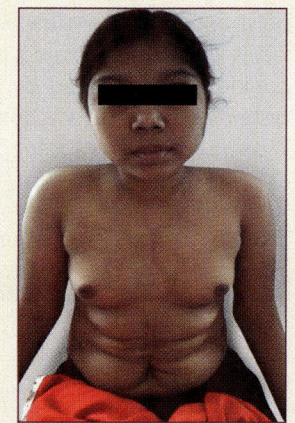

FIG. 1: Breast development after 3 years estrogen replacement.

DISCUSSION

Hemoglobin E-beta thalassemia (HbE/β-thalassemia) is a common variety of hemoglobinopathy in this part of the world. This compound heterozygous state for HbE and β thalassemia is a remarkable heterogenous disease with a presentation ranging from non-transfusion-dependent patients with mild anemia to the severely affected transfusion-dependent patients with devastating iron overload diseases. This girl was on monthly blood transfusions since 18 months of age along with iron chelation therapy. Hypersplenism, as a consequence of splenomegaly, is commonly seen in hemoglobinopathies and splenectomy reduces transfusion requirements. This patient underwent splenectomy at 5 years of age when the transfusion requirement was increased. Repeated blood transfusions cause iron deposition as shown by high serum ferritin levels and leads to many endocrine organ dysfunction. Many of them suffer from poor growth, poor sexual maturation and poor quality of life. Although, the exact mechanism in which iron overload causes tissue damage is not completely understood, oxidative damage by free radicals may affect the pituitary, ovarian follicles, pancreas, and other endocrine organs.

Diabetes mellitus is a major endocrinopathy for patients with hemoglobinopathies. Age, amount of blood transfusion, high ferritin value and family history of diabetes mellitus are the risk factors of diabetes. Apart from iron overload causing β-cell destruction, glucose intolerance and diabetes mellitus among the thalassemic patients may occur from autoimmunity (type 1 diabetes mellitus), genetic insulin resistance (type 2 diabetes mellitus) or insulin resistance secondary to iron-induced liver disease. Both hemoglobinopathies and liver disease, a common consequence of iron overload, can produce false glycosylated hemoglobin (HbA1c) results and hence HbA1c is not suitable for the assessment of long-term blood glucose control. Fructosamine should be considered to monitor glycemic control in patients who have both diabetes and hemoglobinopathies. As fructosamine assessment could not be done in our medical set up, weekly 4 point capillary blood glucose monitoring was carried out in this girl.

Growth and development are often compromised among patients with hemoglobinopathies. Pituitary dysfunction may cause growth failure due to growth hormone deficiency. The expected height for age of the patient was less (SD score-2.5 cm), as assessed by Indian Academy of Pediatrics (IAP) growth charts. The cause of this short stature is often multifactorial and includes iron overload, intensive use of iron chelators, chronic anemia, hypothyroidism, and hypogonadism apart from possible growth hormone deficiency/insufficiency. This patient had chronic anemia, iron overload (serum ferritin of 5612.13 ng/mL), hypogonadism, and received chronic chelation therapy. Her thyroid function was normal and growth hormone study was not done in view of her financial inability to receive growth hormone therapy even if the result came out to be positive. However, her height improved from 141.5 cm to 145.5 cm without any specific therapy, possibly due to improvement in ferritin and correction of hypogonadism.

Delayed puberty in girls, defined by the absence of any breast development at the age of 13 years, is common in hemoglobinopathies and is almost 50–60% among β thalassemia major patients. Ovarian failure is responsible for delayed puberty and may occur due to follicle-stimulating hormone (FSH) and luteinizing hormone (LH) deficiency (hypogonadotropic hypogonadism) or iron deposition in the ovaries itself (hypogonadotropic hypogonadism) or a combination of the above two. This 16-year-old girl had not attained her menarche and had no pubertal development with Tanner stage 1 breast, pubic and axillary hair at the time of presentation. She had ovarian failure as shown by low estrogen level and possibly from pituitary dysfunction (hypogonadotropic hypogonadism) as shown by low FSH and LH levels. Hormone replacement therapy (HRT) in females with hypogonadism may induce puberty and prevent long-term complications such as osteoporosis. However, HRT has risks for thromboembolic disease, cardiovascular events and cancer. Ethinyl estradiol (2.5–5 µg daily) is conventionally recommended in hemoglobinopathies for 18–24 months, followed by estrogen–progesterone combination to induce puberty and regular cyclic bleeding. Estrogen replacement therapy in our patient successfully increased the breast size but did not induce any pubic or axillary hair growth. After 3 years of uninterrupted estrogen replacement therapy, progesterone was added in her regimen to induce regular cyclic bleeding.

Apart from diabetes and hypogonadism, significant proportion of thalassemic patients suffers from other endocrinopathies (especially hypoparathyroidism and hypothyroidism) also. Fortunately, this girl did not have hypoparathyroidism or hypothyroidism. A joint clinic to optimize diabetes, endocrine, and thalassemia care, while supporting patient self-management, is the need of the hour.

Take Home Message

- *Despite early establishment of appropriate chelation therapy, endocrine abnormalities are common complications of hemoglobinopathies.*

SUGGESTED READING

1. Cappellini MD, Cohen A, Eleftheriou A. Guidelines for the Clinical Management of Thalassaemia, 2nd Revised edition. Nicosia: Thalassaemia International Federation; 2008.
2. De Sanctis V, Soliman AT, Elsedfy H, et al. Growth and endocrine disorders in thalassemia: The international network on endocrine complications in thalassemia (I-CET) position statement and guidelines. Indian J Endocrinol Metab. 2013;17(1):8-18.
3. Merchant RH, Shirodkar A, Ahmed J. Evaluation of growth, puberty and endocrine dysfunctions in relation to iron overload in multi transfused Indian thalassemia patients. Indian J Pediatr. 2011;78(6):679-83.

SECTION 4

Diabetes

CASE 1: A Young Ketosis Prone Diabetic

Anirban Mazumdar

CASE HISTORY

A 19-year-old girl presented to the outpatient clinic because of recent detection of high blood sugar. Her past medical history was unremarkable and her mother and maternal grandmother were diabetic. At the time of her diagnosis, she weighed 65 kg with a body mass index (BMI) of 29 kg/m². Physical examination showed acanthosis nigricans; rest of the examination was unremarkable.

Biochemical investigations are summarized in Table 1. Fasting C-peptide level was 3.6 ng/mL indicating adequate beta-cell functional reserve. All these tests supported the diagnosis of type 2 diabetes mellitus (T2DM). She was initially managed with diet, exercise and metformin and 4 months later, her blood sugar levels were consistently controlled with metformin only.

TABLE 1: Biochemical investigation.

Test	Value	Normal range
Fasting plasma glucose	180 mg/dL	70–99
Postprandial plasma glucose	256 mg/dL	70–139
Glycosylated hemoglobin	8.4%	4–5.6
Serum creatinine	0.76 mg/dL	0.6–1.2
Thyroid function	Normal	–
Fasting C-peptide level	3.6 ng/mL	0.51–2.72

She did well until 1 week ago, when she noted polyuria, polydipsia and rising fingerstick glucose values, higher than 300 mg/dL. She was presented in the emergency room of the hospital with vomiting, symptoms of dehydration and altered mental status. She denied any fever, chills, cough, abdominal pain or dysuria. Laboratory tests revealed severe hyperglycemia (random 567 mg/dL) with no evidence of acute infection, renal or liver dysfunction. The arterial pH was 7.1 (normal 7.35–7.45), anion gap was high, serum bicarbonate (8 mmol/L) was low, urine was positive for ketones (acetoacetate) and she was diagnosed with diabetic ketoacidosis (DKA) (Fig. 1). During her hospital stay, the fasting C-peptide level was rechecked and it was undetectable (less than 0.5 ng/mL). She received standard treatment for DKA with IV fluids and insulin and recovered uneventfully. She was discharged on the 5th hospital day on a basal-bolus

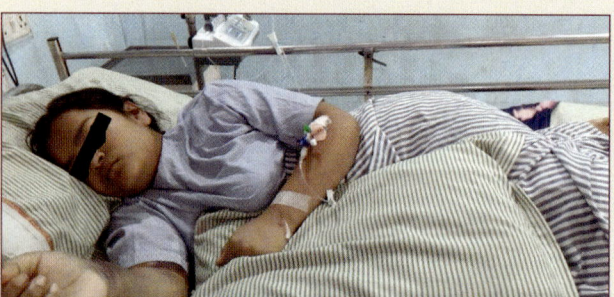

FIG. 1: Young and obese patient with diabetic ketoacidosis.

insulin regimen. She remained stable on basal-bolus regimen, but gained 3 kg weight in 4 months. Beta-cell functional reserve was reassessed and fasting C-peptide level had come up to 2.8 ng/mL. She was further evaluated for autoantibodies to glutamic acid decarboxylase (GAD) 65 and islet tyrosine phosphatase 2 antibodies (IA-A2) and both were absent. An attempt was made to switch her to oral antidiabetic agents in lieu of her repeat C-peptide level of 2.8 ng/mL. She was started on glimiperide 2 mg daily and metformin 1,000 mg twice daily and insulin was gradually discontinued. Over next 6 months glimiperide was also stopped. For the last 6 months she is on metformin 1,000 mg twice daily only without any further episode of DKA and her last HbA1c 1 month ago was 6.8%.

DISCUSSION

Diabetic ketoacidosis was once considered a hallmark feature of type 1 diabetes mellitus (T1DM) and was used in clinical practice to differentiate it from the more common T2DM. However, some patients present with DKA or unprovoked ketosis, despite lacking the classic autoimmune markers of T1DM. These ketosis prone individuals with negative autoantibodies are frequently associated with Human leukocyte antigen (HLA) class II DRB1*03 and/or DRB1*04 and this is commonly referred to as Flatbush diabetes mellitus.

This 19-year-old obese girl with positive family history of diabetes had no evidence of beta cell autoimmunity, had signs of insulin resistance (acanthosis nigricans). She was initially managed with oral hypoglycemic agents and presented with DKA. She did fine on an attempt to switch her to oral agents 4 months after recovery from DKA when beta cells had recovered from glucose toxicity. She was diagnosed with flatbush diabetes mellitus. However, we could not check HLA typing in our medical set-up.

Flatbush diabetes is a unique form of diabetes commonly described among African-American patients with DKA as the initial manifestation without any identifiable precipitating cause for DKA. This atypical presentation has also been reported in Asian countries including India and is being recognized increasingly worldwide. The pathophysiologic mechanisms involved are unknown. Severe impairment of both insulin secretion and insulin action are the most dominating pathophysiologies at presentation. The relation between this transient severe impairment of insulin secretion and HLA class II antigen is largely unknown. Aggressive diabetes management improve both beta-cell function and insulin sensitivity leading to discontinuation of insulin therapy within a few months as demonstrated in our case.

TABLE 2: Classification of ketosis-prone diabetes.

GAD antibodies or IA-2 autoantibodies	β-cell functional reserve	HLA antigen	Diagnosis
A+	B–	HLA-DR3 and/or HLA-DR4	KPD type 1A: Autoimmune Type 1 diabetes
A–	B–	Nil	KPD type 1B: Nonautoimmune Type 1 diabetes
A+	B+	HLA-DR3	KPD type 2A: LADA
A–	B+	HLA-DR3 and HLA-DR4	KPD type 2B: Flatbush diabetes

(GAD: glutamic acid decarboxylase; HLA: human leukocyte antigen; IA-A2: islet tyrosine phosphatase 2 antibodies; KPD: ketosis-prone diabetes; LADA: late onset autoimmune diabetes in adults)

Ketosis-prone diabetes (KPD) is heterogeneous and Flatbush diabetes is one variety of KPD. They are classified into four groups (Table 2), based on the presence of GAD antibodies or IA-2 autoantibodies (A+ or A–) and β-cell functional reserve/C-peptide response (β+ or β–). KPD type 1A is the classic autoimmune T1DM accompanied by permanent and complete beta cell failure along with serologic markers of islets cell autoimmunity (A+, B–). KPD type 1B is the nonautoimmune variety T1DM with permanent and complete beta-cell failure, but lacking the serologic markers of islet cell autoimmunity (A–, B–). KPD type 2A is the late onset autoimmune diabetes in adults (LADA) with preserved beta-cell function at the time of diagnosis and has serologic markers of islet cell autoimmunity (A+, B+). KPD type 2B is flatbush diabetes where beta-cell function is preserved and serologic markers of islet cell autoimmunity are lacking (A–, B+). Hence, KPD comprises at least four etiologically distinct subtypes and is separable by GAD/IA-2 autoantibodies, HLA genotype and C-peptide response (β-cell reserve). The cause of β-cell dysfunction that leads to DKA among the flatbush diabetes and nonautoimmune T1DM is largely unknown and one or multiple novel, nonautoimmune mechanisms are likely to underlie the cause.

Take Home Message

- Evaluation of autoantibodies and C-peptide in young diabetic patients are often required to categorize the type of diabetes.

SUGGESTED READING

1. Lebovitz HE, Banerji MA. Ketosis-Prone Diabetes (Flatbush Diabetes): an Emerging Worldwide Clinically Important Entity. Curr Diab Rep. 2018;18(11):120.
2. Maldonado M, Hampe CS, Gaur LK. Ketosis-prone diabetes: dissection of a heterogeneous syndrome using an immunogenetic and beta-cell functional classification, prospective analysis, and clinical outcomes. J Clin Endocrinol Metab. 2003;88:5090-8.

CASE 2
Common Problem...Where Lies the Solution?
Biswajit Ghoshdastidar

CASE HISTORY

A 78-year-old female, known type 2 diabetes mellitus with past history NHL (non-Hodgkin's lymphoma-received chemotherapy and six cycles of radiotherapy), was admitted with sudden change in behavior associated with poor glycemic control.

General and systemic examination was unremarkable. However, she had profound hallucinatory and delusional symptoms and was difficult to manage in the ward. Routine hematological and biochemistry ruled out hyponatremia, hypercalcemia and sepsis or hepatic encephalopathy. Contrast-enhanced CT brain ruled out any NHL recurrence and revealed "age-related cerebral atrophy", which obviously does not explain her symptoms. Psychiatric assessment revealed acute psychosis in the background of severe depression and psychotropic medication was started. Response was dramatic and her orientation returned completely and went home with a reasonably clear state of mind.

Following is her inpatients glycemic profile with HbA1c as high as 16% (Tables 1 and 2).

She had been on glimepiride 2 mg and metformin 1,000 mg daily at home. Blood glucose values in-patients ranged from 300 mg/dL to 550 mg/dL requiring minimal dose of insulin during first 2 days, which was managed with supplemental insulin; however, her glycemic control rapidly returned to normal level requiring minimal dose of insulin in the controlled hospital environment. She went home after 1 week with a gliptin and metformin and advice of home monitoring of blood glucose. Her husband died 2 years

TABLE 1: Poor glycemic control (the only striking feature).

Test	Value	Normal range
SGOT (UV with P5P) V	24 U/L	14–36
SGPT (UV with P5P) V	26 U/L	9–52
Alkaline phosphatase (PNPP) V	134 U/L	38–126
Total bilirubin (DDS) V	0.6 mg/dL	0.2–1.3
Total protien (BEP) V	7.3 mg/dL	6.3–8.2
Albumin (BCG) V	4.2 mg/dL	3.5–6.0
Globulin (Calculated) V	3.1 mg/dL	2.8–3.2
Ratio (A:G) (Calculated) V	1.38	–
Gamma G T (GGPN) V	11 U/L	12–43
Urea (Urease) V	28.48 mg/dL	14.98–36.38
Creatinine (IFCC) V	0.92 mg/dL	0.52–1.04
Uric acid (Uricase) V	4.31 mg/dL	2.5–6.2
LDH total (L>P) V	175 µL	120–246
Glycosylated hemoglobin	16.0%	<6.0 nondiabetic <7.0 well controlled >8.0 poor controlled

ago and she has been living alone since then. She has a daughter, living close by, but too tied up with her own family and visits her only occasionally. She reluctantly agreed to visit her mother once a week to check her blood sugar.

Now it is obvious that the high HbA1c is a reflection of her completely erratic lifestyle and withdrawal of antidiabetic medication for many months, which remained undetected because of very poor social support and perhaps inadequate awareness about mental health among healthcare providers and the caregivers. With a proper infrastructure, this unfortunate situation leading to unnecessary hospitalization could have been prevented.

TABLE 2: Rapid restoration of blood glucose level in hospital environment even without insulin at the end.

Date	Time	Capillary blood glucose (mg/dL)
24/01/19	2 PM	308
	5 PM	292
	7 PM	558
	10 PM	338
25/01/19	7 PM	125
	12 PM	80
	2 PM	110
	7 PM	120
	10 PM	140
26/01/19	12:30 AM	67
	2 AM	124
	5 AM	90
	7 PM	155
	12 PM	125
	7 PM	206
	10 PM	272
27/01/19	2 AM	152
	5 AM	142
	7 PM	179
	12 PM	198

DISCUSSION

Psychiatric illnesses among diabetic subjects are not uncommon and pose a special challenge to physicians, not only in resource-deprived countries but in developed world too, in community as well as hospital in-patient mainly due to lack of structured training in the diabetes team and poor linkage with psychiatry team.

British psychiatrists and diabetes societies have drawn up a joint guideline (Diabetes UK Position Statement) in 2018 for managing diabetes with psychiatrist disorder in in-patients settings (www.diabetes.org.uk/joint-british-diabetis-society and http://abcd.care/joint-british-diabetis-society-jbds-inpatient-care-group). This guideline, interestingly has incorporated a few community based preventive management as well. Some of the points are being highlighted here:

1. *Older people (>65 years)*: All with diabetes mellitus should be screened and be assessed for cognitive impairment, depression, psychosis and alcohol use, if there are concerns that such conditions may hinder diabetes self-management or may have contributed to the hospital admission
2. All psychiatric patients in community should be screened for diabetes
3. All psychiatric patients with known diabetes should have medicines to be reviewed to ensure use of antidiabetics with low risk of hypoglycemia. Those requiring insulin should have doses regularly reviewed
4. *Dementia care*:

Four-step approach			
Proactive screening for diabetes	Symptom alleviation + assessment of complication	Risk minimization	Palliative care approach in advance dementia

5. *Diabetes care*:

Four-step approach			
Increase awareness and screening for dementia	Managing cognitive deficit	Minimize therapy risk	Palliative care approach in advance dementia

6. All diabetic ketoacidosis should be screened for psychiatric disorder (using formal ICD-10) and also psychological distress
7. Training and educational needs of caregivers in the management of diabetes and dementia
8. *Inpatients in acute hospital setting*:

Three-step approach		
All DKA episodes	Any evidence of self-herm	Multiple comorbidities
↓	↓	↓
Screen for psychological factors	1. Screen for suicidal ideation 2. Supervise self-administration of insulin	Multidisciplinary team meeting to support self-management and care
↓		
Psychiatric referrals where cause not explained by medical factors		

9. *Substance misuse and learning disability*: They have higher risk of amputation and diabetes related complication

Three-step approach		
Create a registry	Monitor glycosylated hemoglobin, blood pressure, dyslipidemia	Weigh benefit of psychotropic medication against the risk of obesity

10. Eating disorder and type 1 diabetes mellitus—A very complex problem.

Research and piloting of innovations in models of care are needed to improve care for this group.

> **Take Home Message**
> - An integrated mind–body approach to diabetes (both inpatients and outpatients) within the constraints of economic and manpower resource is a need of the hour in our country. A special task force should be employed to generate a country (India) specific guideline and raise awareness among the healthcare providers.

SUGGESTED READING

1. Schmidt CB, Potter van Loon BJ, Vergouwen ACM, et al. Systematic review and meta-analysis of psychological interventions in people with diabetes and elevated diabetes-distress. Diabet Med. 2018;35:1157-72.
2. Price HC, Ismail K. Royal College of Psychiatrists Liaison Faculty & Joint British Diabetes Societies (JBDS): guidelines for the management of diabetes in adults and children with psychiatric disorders in inpatient settings. Diabet Med. 2018;35:997-1004.

CASE 3: A Diabetic with Infected Hand

Anirban Mazumdar

CASE HISTORY

A 46-year-old man with recently detected diabetes, presented with painful gangrene in his left thumb (Figs. 1 and 2). A needle had pricked his thumb 7 days ago. He had no history suggestive of peripheral neuropathy and all modalities of sensation in both upper and lower limbs were intact. He had no intermittent claudication or ulcers in feet. He was a nonsmoker and not an intravenous drug abuser. He was an occasional drinker for past 5 years. On presentation at our hospital, he was normotensive and hemodynamically stable with normal radial pulse on both sides. He had very high (580 mg/dL) capillary plasma glucose during presentation.

The following evaluations were done at the time of presentation (Table 1).

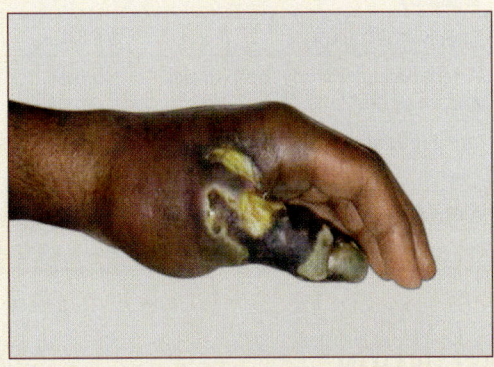

FIG. 1: Ulceration and gangrene in left thumb.

He underwent aggressive debridement and surgical amputation of the thumb under cover of intravenous antibiotics (ceftriaxone 1 g 12 hourly and metronidazole 500 mg 8 hourly) and insulin. Culture of debrided tissue revealed *Staphylococcus aureus*, *Klebsiella pneumoniae* and *Pseudomonas aeruginosa* strain. The wound healed gradually over 2 weeks time with proper sensitive antibiotics and insulin therapy.

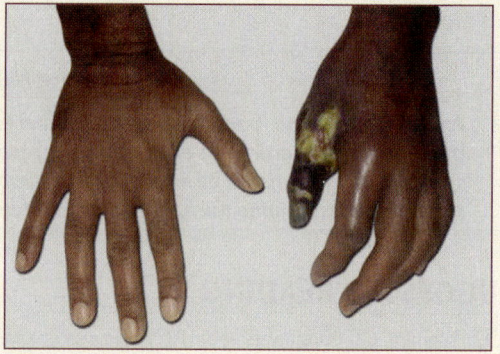

FIG. 2: Gangrene in left thumb with spreading inflammation proximally and unaffected right hand.

TABLE 1: Laboratory parameters at the time of presentation.

Investigations	Results	Normal range
Hemoglobin	11.7 g/dL	12–16
Total leukocyte count	21,700/cumm	3,500–11,000
Platelet	320,000/cumm	150,000–450,000
Erythrocyte sedimentation rate	63 mm/h	0–22
C-reactive protein	38 mg/L	Below 3.0
Fasting plasma glucose	267 mg/dL	70–99
Postprandial plasma glucose	549 mg/dL	70–139
Glycosylated hemoglobin	11.7%	3.6–5.6
Serum creatinine	0.8 mg/dL	0.6–1.2
Liver function test	Normal	
Immunofluorescent antinuclear antibody	Negative	Less than or equal to 1:40
Rheumatoid factor	6.5 IU/mL	Less than 15
Arterial doppler study (both upper and lower limbs)	Normal	
Urine routine	Glucose: present RBC: absent	
X-ray	No bony abnormality	

DISCUSSION

Infection and gangrene in diabetics commonly involve lower limbs and hand infection is less recognized than foot infections. Hand involvement may be due to associated systemic sclerosis, trauma, connective tissue disorders, vasculitic disorders, as a part of tropical diabetes hand syndrome (TDHS) but rarely from upper limb arterio-occlusive disease as a macrovascular complication of diabetes. Normal renal function with absent red blood cells in urine, normal liver function test and normal platelet count are indicative of lack of systemic involvement in our case. Absent rheumatoid factor and negative immunofluorescent antinuclear antibody (FANA) are suggestive of absence of connective tissue disorders. Arterial Doppler study was done to evaluate any upper limb arterio-occulsive disease. The hand infection and gangrene in this diabetic subject was without any evidence of upper limb arterio-occulsive disease, systemic sclerosis, connective tissue disorders or vasculitic disorders. This presentation of diabetic hand is a rare clinical presentation and known as TDHS.

The TDHS is a specific acute symptom complex found in diabetic patients in tropics. It usually follows minor trauma to the hand and leads to a fulminant hand sepsis with gangrene, as seen in our case. The antecedent minor trauma is often as trivial as scratches or insect bites and presentation to the hospital is often delayed due to the unawareness of the potential seriousness. The severe consequences of TDHS are amputation, permanent disability and death. Immediate appropriate antimicrobial therapy is the key to success. The swab cultures yield polymicrobial flora in the majority (probably because of contamination) whereas culture of tissue biopsy specimens mostly yield a single bacterial species and thus is a better approach. However, even culture of tissue biopsy yielded polymicrobial flora in our case and required combined antibiotic therapy. The infection is often more extensive than suspected and prompt aggressive wound management with incision, debridement and drainage of the wound is required. Observation, local wound care and oral antibiotic therapy are not acceptable approach in TDHS. Through the majority of reported cases have been from various parts of the African continent, TDHS has been reported among patients in India also. Early recognition by patients, prompt medical attention and proper glycemic control might reduce the disability and death from this condition.

Take Home Message

- A minor trauma to the hand of a diabetic may lead to a progressive fulminant hand sepsis with gangrene.

SUGGESTED READING

1. Abbas ZG, Archibald LK. Tropical diabetic hand syndrome. Epidemiology, pathogenesis, and management. Am J Clin Dermatol. 2005;6(1):21-8.
2. Nthumba P, Cavadas PC, Landin L. The tropical diabetic hand syndrome: a surgical perspective. Ann Plast Surg. 2013;70(1):42-6.

CASE 4: Advanced Diabetic Nephropathy without Diabetic Retinopathy

Debmalya Sanyal

CASE HISTORY

A 40-year-old male from Bangladesh with hypertension (HTN) and end-stage renal disease (ESRD) due to chronic glomerulonephritis underwent renal allograft transplantation. The patient developed new onset diabetes after transplantation (NODAT). He had hypertension and was on multiple antihypertensive drugs. He had diabetic peripheral neuropathy (DPN). The patient had a poor follow-up, 7 years later his eGFR dropped to 38 with ACR of 178. Renal biopsy of transplanted kidney showed classic nodular glomerulosclerosis (KW lesion) indicating diabetic nephropathy. Diabetes was poorly controlled with HbA1c of 10.2; uncontrolled HTN—176/100, FBS—200, PPBS—289, eGFR—11, ACR—2534, TC—300, LDL—140, 1 year later—ESRD—he had repeat renal allograft transplantation. He had no evidence of diabetic retinopathy (up to two microaneurysms in each side) on direct and indirect ophthalmoscopic examination. Immediate preoperative fundal photograph (Figs. 1 and 2) showed no evidence of diabetic retinopathy (DR). The patient's father died of chronic kidney disease due to diabetes without any retinopathy.

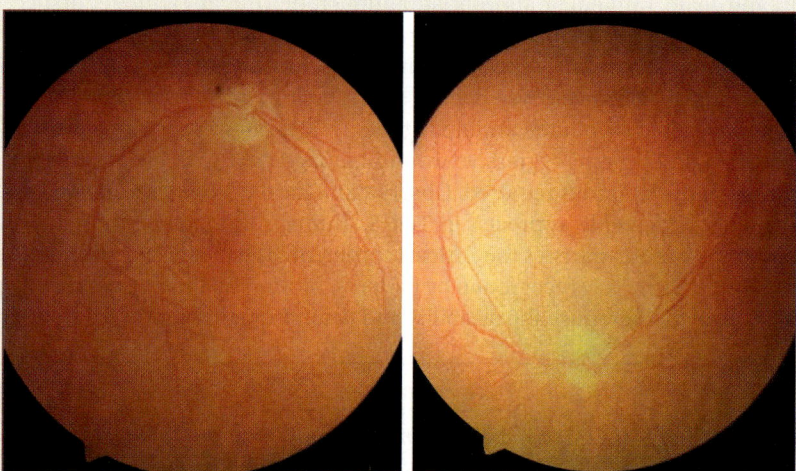

FIG. 1: Fundal photograph showing no evidence of diabetic retinopathy.

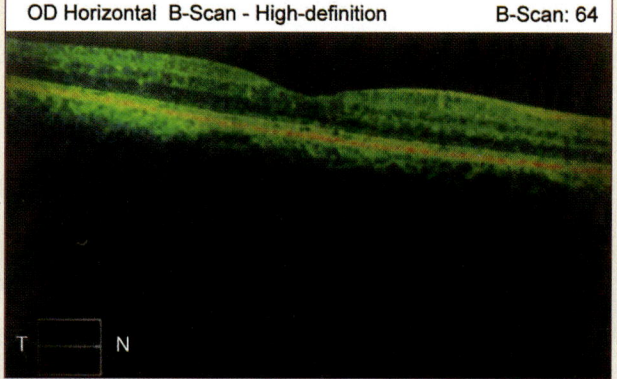

FIG. 2: OCT: no abnormality.

DISCUSSION

There is generally a concordance between eye and renal complications in patients with DM. Though some studies have demonstrated the presence of severe retinopathy without nephropathy, the reverse, i.e. overt nephropathy without retinopathy is rare. Renal retinal relationship in type 2 diabetes mellitus (T2DM) may not be helpful for clinical diagnosis of DN. One-third of T2DM patients with renal biopsy—demonstrated diabetic glomerulopathy do not have retinopathy. DN found in 50% of patients without DR and lack of retinopathy is a poor predictor of nondiabetic kidney disease. In a study, advanced nephropathy was present in 5 of the 122 (4.1%) patients without retinopathy and no special clinical features distinguished the patients who were regarded as having possible advanced nephropathy without retinopathy. For patients with only DR, incidence increased as DM duration increased, for DR and overt nephropathy incidence appeared to be closely related to levels of HbA1c. The Atherosclerosis Risk in Communities (ARIC) Study showed that poor glycemic control in diabetes increase risk of incident CKD even in absence of albuminuria and retinopathy. Visit-to-visit systolic blood pressure variability is an independent predictor of development and progression of DN, but not retinopathy, in T2DM patients. Recent studies demonstrate that an insertion/deletion of polymorphism of different genes is associated with diabetic complications. Genotype II of the angiotensin-converting enzyme gene is a marker for a decreased risk of DN but not for DR. In Chinese subjects, XbaI (2) allele of *GLUT1* gene might be a genetic marker of noninsulin-dependent diabetes mellitus with DN, and this genetic susceptibility is independent of retinopathy.

Take Home Message

- There is well-recognized association between retinopathy and nephropathy, in which nephropathy without retinopathy is rare but retinopathy without nephropathy is common. The standard medical opinion is that DN in the absence of DR should trigger a search for nondiabetic renal disease. It is generally recognized that DR can exist in the absence of DN, but DN, especially ESRD is almost always associated with DR. The fact that microvascular complications in retina and kidney can occur in isolation suggest the existence of specific organ-related pathogenetic factors. Microvascular complications of the kidney do not always spillover to the retina. This suggests that the etiopathogenesis of the two complications are distinct from each other. It is also possible that some individuals with DN and ESRD are genetically protected from DR. Thus, there can be discordance between retinopathy and nephropathy may be present independent of each other and all clinicians should be actively vigilant about independent existence of each complications of diabetes.

SUGGESTED READING

1. Kanauchi M, Kawano T, Uyama H, Shiiki H, Dohi K. Discordance between retinopathy and nephropathy in type 2 diabetes. Nephron. 1998;80:171-4.
2. Marre M, Bernadet P, Gallois Y, et al. Relationships between angiotensin I converting enzyme gene polymorphism, plasma levels, and diabetic retinal and renal complications. Diabetes. 1994;43(3):384-8.
3. Sanyal D, Chatterjee S. Advanced diabetic nephropathy with "Clean" eyes: An extreme phenotype. Indian J Endocr Metab. 2018;22:274-6.

CASE 5

Diabetes Mellitus

Debasis Maji

CASE HISTORY

Patient A

A 10-year-old boy of Class IV was brought to the emergency of a subdivisional hospital in the evening from a nearby village of South 24 Parganas, West Bengal. He was complaining of drowsiness for 2 days and passage of roundworm through mouth as well as in stool for last 1 week. There was nausea, but no vomiting or diarrhea.

He was afebrile, pulse rate: 110 beats/min, BP: 90/60 mm Hg, abdomen: irregular palpable ill-defined, nontender, movable swelling noticed, liver/spleen not palpable, there was no ascites. CVS—no abnormality, CNS—the boy was drowsy but responding to verbal questions and no neurodeficit was noticed. A diagnosis of roundworm toxicity was made. He was admitted under a pediatrician. IV dextrose saline drip started and a tablet of albendazole was given by Ryle's tube. All attention was given to the roundworm infestation and his clinical condition was thought to be due to roundworm infestation.

Next morning he became more drowsy, the detailed history was taken from the mother and it was revealed that for last 2 months he felt weak after coming from school in the afternoon and was becoming thin in spite of good appetite.

On examination, apart from the findings of the previous evening, he was found to have gross dehydration (sunken eyes and loss of elasticity of skin).

Laboratory reports are summarized in Table 1. Urine R/E–sugar ++++, acetone+++: No pus cells, no RBC.

A diagnosis of diabetic ketoacidosis (DKA) was considered and he was put on standard regimen of management of DKA with adequate IV fluid, IV KCl, IV insulin injection, antibiotic, hourly measurement of blood sugar and vital signs. Over the next 3 days, the boy gradually recovered from DKA and blood sugar came down to the normal range. He was given oral feed and put on basal-bolus regimen (i.e. rapid acting insulin before breakfast, lunch and dinner, injection glargine at bedtime). Over the next 4 days the parents were educated on insulin injection, dietary regulation, monitoring of

TABLE 1: Laboratory reports.

Test	Value
Hemoglobin	14 g%
Total leukocyte count	14,000/mm^3
Polymorphonuclear leukocyte	70%
Fasting blood glucose	610 mg/dL
Urea	48 mg/dL
Serum creatinine	1.15 mg/dL
Serum bicarbonate	10 mEq/L
Serum sodium	136 mEq/L
Serum potassium	4.3 mEq/L

blood sugar, tackling hypoglycemia and sick day rules. During his hospital stay he passed 67 roundworms with stool and his abdominal lumps disappeared. He was discharged 7 days after admission with no complaints.

Patient B

A 48-year-old female had type 1 diabetes mellitus (T1DM) for the last 26 years. She complained of repeated attacks of hypoglycemia, in spite of close monitoring of her blood sugar several times a day. She was on basal bolus regimen (injection actrapid 10 units before breakfast, lunch and dinner and injection lantus 12 units at bedtime). She got hypoglycemia attacks mostly during early morning and late afternoon. During her hypoglycemia attacks, she felt dizziness, headache and heaviness of head for few minutes. After this she became unconscious and fell down. She does not feel palpitation, tachycardia, trembling of body or sweating. A glass of glucose water is kept always ready when she is at home. When she goes outside, she keeps glucose powder in her bag and she carries her identity card with her, mentioning about her disease, about her hypoglycemia episodes and directions about what to do in such situations. She has very rarely had hospital admission for her hypoglycemia attacks, because her family members and employer are very much aware about the hypoglycemic attacks. She is very well educated type 1 diabetic patient and takes part as a diabetic educator in group therapy of other type 1 diabetic patients in a diabetic clinic.

Several occasions she tried to adjust the insulin dose, but reduction of insulin dose lead to hyperglycemia and slight increase will lead to hypoglycemia. She is very active and tries hard to maintain her blood sugar under control so that she can prevent microvascular complications of diabetes. She does not have retinopathy, nephropathy or neuropathy. She is well educated about diabetes control, its complications, but hypoglycemia episodes continued to trouble her and her family members. Yearly total body check up shows the following reports for last 5 years.

The patient complained of nausea and vomiting on three occasions over the last 3 months. She also complained of darkening of her complexion. Serum cortisol was done and found to be low (3 µg/dL). ACTH stimulations test confirmed adrenal insufficiency (basal cortisol 3 µg/mL and after ACTH stimulation 3.3 µg/dL). She was put on wysolone 5 mg in the morning and 2.5 mg in the evening. Last 6 months her hypoglycemia episodes have become negligible, weakness and nausea have gone. She is now asymptomatic (Table 2).

TABLE 2: Stable glucose parameters of patient.

Fasting	Lunch		Dinner	
	Before	After	Before	After
106	118	226	102	212
122	168		148	
118	136	272	170	242
132	146		118	
118	126	232	102	222
112	136		118	282
128	132	280	106	242

Note: Blood sugar in mg/dL.

Patient C

A 14-year-old male type 1 diabetic patient complained of late night disturbance of sleep off and on. Most of the time it was associated with nightmares. He has been diagnosed to have TIDM for last 1 year. He is now studying in class VIII. In class VII he had lot of problems in adjusting with regular insulin injections and frequent blood sugar check as advised by the doctor. He became irregular in school due to difficulties in taking regular insulin injection especially at school premises. The fear of taking insulin injection in front of others was psychologically upsetting for him. He was nervous and anxious. After regular visit to doctor's clinic every month, now he takes his own injection and follows doctor's advice. Initially he was taking premixed insulin twice daily (injection mixtard 30/70 16 units before breakfast and 10 units before dinner). His blood sugar used to fluctuate with periods of high blood sugar (>200 mg/dL). As he is familiar with insulin injection and he now does not mind taking insulin injection at school in front of his friends, his doctor has put him on basal bolus regimen (i.e. 6 units actrapid before breakfast, lunch and dinner, injection lantus 14 units at bedtime. His blood sugar is now within satisfactory range (Table 3).

Parents were happy to see that the blood sugar control became much better and doctor was much happy during his last clinic visit. But the sleep disturbance and fearful nightmares which the boy was having almost regularly worried the parents. They were thinking of taking the boy to a psychiatrist. Before doing that they consulted their treating physician who advised them to do a blood sugar test at 3 o'clock night for two consecutive days it came out to be 34 mg/dL and 52 mg/dL.

Doctor advised to reduce the dose of injection lantus by 2 units at bedtime and the dose of actrapid before dinner by 2 units. Next 2 days the 3 a.m. blood sugar measured was 98 mg/dL and 101 mg/dL respectively and he stopped having nightmares and slept comfortably throughout night.

So the whole problem was due to hypoglycemia attack in the early hours of the morning. Which is not uncommon in type 1 diabetic patient who tries to keep the blood sugar under tight control daytime. There is normal dip in blood sugar during late night hours which was aggravated in this patient and the anxiety and nightmares are due to the sympathetic system overactivity due to hypoglycemia.

TABLE 3: Patient C's blood glucose chart.

Fasting	Lunch		Dinner	
	Before	After	Before	After
100	98	146	98	152
98	102	150	102	148
102	106	156	100	146
106	101	148	98	161
100	111	152	102	152
98	98	162	98	149
102	98	148	101	152

Note: Blood sugar in mg/dL.

Take Home Messages

- **Patient A:** Most important clinical sign of diabetic ketoacidosis is dehydration. This patient had dehydration without any diarrhea or vomiting. Roundworm infestation in this case is a coincidental event and it is very common in villages. Currently, roundworm toxicity is not recognized as a disease. T1DM in India is not common in India as compared to western countries. However, 15% of T1DM cases first present with DKA while the remaining 85% cases present with polyuria, polydipsia, polyphagia and weakness. On many occasions we may miss the diagnosis, like in this case where all attention was given to roundworm infestation when attention should have been given to the severe dehydration the boy had
- **Patient B:** The T1DM due to its autoimmune mechanism may be associated with other autoimmune disease particularly autoimmune thyroid disorders. In this case it was adrenal insufficiency, which is rare. Clinical presentation in this case was with hypoglycemia which is quite a common symptom in T1DM patients
- **Patient C:** Type 1 diabetic patient, whoever tries to go for tight blood sugar control, will experience hypoglycemia episodes. The treating physician should remain aware of rare hypoglycemia manifestations, as seen in this case.

SUGGESTED READING

1. Kalra S, Mukherjee JJ, Venkataraman S, et al. Hypoglycemia: The neglected complication. Indian J Endocrinol Metab. 2013;17(5):819-34.
2. Lambert PHL, Jourdan PM. Human Ascariasis: Diagnostics Update. Curr Trop Med Rep. 2015;2(4): 189-200.
3. Samaan NA. Hypoglycemia secondary to endocrine deficiencies. Endocrinol Metab Clin North Am. 1989;18(1):145-54.

CASE 6: Diabetes and the Breast
Kalyan Kumar Gangopadhyay

CASE HISTORY

A 38-year-old lady was referred to the surgeon for assessment of a breast mass. She had type 1 diabetes mellitus (T1DM) since the age of 21 years and had background of diabetic retinopathy. She had a breast lump in her right breast 4 years ago the biopsy of which revealed fibrocystic changes. She was increasingly worried that it might turn out to have a malignant pathology.

Her medications included insulin lispro 6 units, 10 units and 18 units before breakfast, lunch and dinner respectively and insulin glargine 28 units daily. Her HbA1c was 11.6%.

Examination revealed a 3 cm firm but mobile lump in the upper lateral quadrant of the right breast. Ultrasound failed to reveal any clear abnormality.

She proceeded to have a lumpectomy. The lump measured 4 × 3 × 2.8 cm and appeared irregular on macroscopic examination. On microscopic examination (Fig. 1), there appeared to be atrophic changes around some of the ducts and lobules. There was a patchy but brisk lymphocytic infiltrate surrounding those ducts and lobules along with evidence of fibrosis. Hence the diagnosis was given as lymphocytic mastitis or diabetic mastopathy.

She remained free of any breast lumps till about 4 years of follow-up.

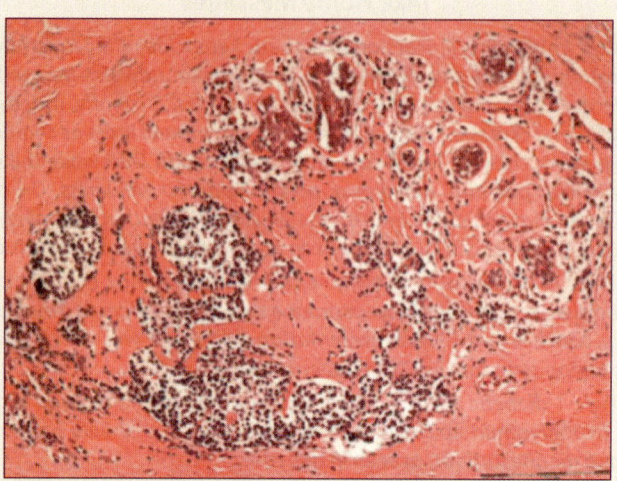

FIG. 1: Microscopic findings of the lesion of this patient. Note the lymphocytic infiltration, destruction and loss of some of the terminal ducts and dense fibrosis.

DISCUSSION

Prevalence

The association between this type of breast lesion and diabetes was first described as late as in 1984. Although the exact prevalence is unknown, it accounts for less than 1% of all benign breast pathologies, but may be present in 1–13% of women with type 1 diabetes mellitus (T1DM) in the reproductive age. The association between diabetic mastopathy and type 2 diabetes mellitus (T2DM) is weaker than that of T1DM. Although the western literature suggests that diabetic mastopathy occurs more in T1DM than in T2DM, studies from southeast Asia revealed that diabetic mastopathy occurred more in T2DM and more so in those T2DM who were on insulin.

Pathogenesis

Although the exact pathogenesis is not completely understood, the most plausible theory is that the poorly controlled diabetes leads to increased accumulation of glycosylation end products which, act as a neoantigen, triggers an autoimmune response with B cell proliferation and antibody production with consequent cytokine release, which then leads to extracellular matrix expansion.

Clinical and Laboratory Features

Clinically, it presents as a single or multiple ill-defined firm to hard mass, which are not tender. This often raises the suspicion of malignancy.

Mammography usually reveals an irregular focal mass of very dense breast tissue. Ultrasound may show an irregular area of a hypoechoic mass. However mastopathy and malignancy cannot be distinguished with certainty using the current imaging techniques.

TABLE 1: Constellation of findings based on which the diagnosis of diabetic mastopathy may be made.

No.	Clinical, radiological and pathological features
1	Premenopausal women with long-standing diabetes
2	Hard, nontender, palpable breast mass clinically suspicious for malignancy
3	Mammography—increased density but unable to localize the mass
4	Ultrasound—fails to identify a solid or cystic mass
5	Excisional or core biopsy—dense keloidal fibrosis with periductal, perivascular, perilobular lymphocytic infiltrate

Microscopic examination reveals periductal, perilobular or perivascular lymphocytic infiltrate along with keloidal fibrosis. The complete constellation of lymphocytic lobulitis, ductitis, vasculitis and keloidal fibrosis is not present in chronic mastitis of nondiabetic individuals making this peculiar to patients with diabetes.

Table 1 shows the clinical features based on which the diagnosis of diabetic mastopathy may be made.

Management

The diagnosis can be made on core biopsy thereby avoiding unnecessary extensive surgical procedures. Treatment with excisional biopsy is sufficient for unilateral disease. For follow-up routine self-examination and annual mammography is recommended. About 30–60% of the cases may recur, either on the ipsilateral, contralateral or both breasts. Hence asymptomatic histologically confirmed diabetic mastopathy may be managed conservatively. Diabetic mastopathy has not been linked to further development of breast malignancy.

Take Home Messages

- *Diabetic mastopathy is an uncommon benign fibrotic disease affecting women with long-standing diabetes*
- *Although it may be difficult to differentiate from breast carcinoma both clinically and radiologically, it has characteristic of histological features*
- *There is a high risk of recurrence after surgical excision*
- *There is no increase in risk of breast carcinoma*
- *Knowledge of this clinical pathology combined with core needle biopsy would lead to avoidance of surgical excision which can lead to recurrence.*

SUGGESTED READING

1. Shrikrishnapalasuriyar N, Atkinson M, Kalhan A, et al. Diabetic mastopathy: a diagnostic challenge. Br J Diabetes. 2018;18:32-4.
2. Suvannarerg V, Claimon T, Sitthinamsuwan P, et al. Clinical, mammographic, and ultrasonographic characteristics of diabetic mastopathy: A case series. Clin Imaging. 2019;53:204-9.
3. Tomaszewski JE, Brooks JS, Hick D, et al. Diabetic mastopathy: a distinctive clinicopathological entity. Hum Pathol. 1992;23:780-6.

CASE 7: Cellulitis Mimic in Diabetes

Kalyan Kumar Gangopadhyay

CASE HISTORY

A 60-year-old lady with type 2 diabetes mellitus (T2DM) of 15 years duration and hypertension presented with progressive pain and swelling of left thigh for 2 weeks. She did not complain of any fever. She had received courses of several antibiotics prior to presentation at our set-up without any benefit.

Her body temperature was 36.9°C. Examination of the local area revealed diffuse swelling over the anterolateral aspect of the upper third of the left thigh with erythema and tenderness. She had proliferative diabetic retinopathy. There was no evidence of local hyperthermia.

Her WBC count was 15,000/μL, CRP: 22 mg/L, eGFR: 30 mL/min/1.73 m^2 and HbA1c was 10.7%.

Ultrasound doppler of the limb did not reveal any features of vascular pathology. Muscle striations were however reportedly lost. Tissue edema was present, but interestingly there was no evidence of any purulent collection. Contrast-enhanced images showed heterogeneous contrast enhancement of the anterior compartment muscles of the left thigh with hyperintense areas of normal muscle, and contained intramuscularly, well-delineated nonenhancing hypointense areas suggestive of necrosis (Figs. 1A to C). This picture of muscular necrosis on the background of her tell-tale clinical features helped to establish the diagnosis of diabetic myonecrosis (DMN).

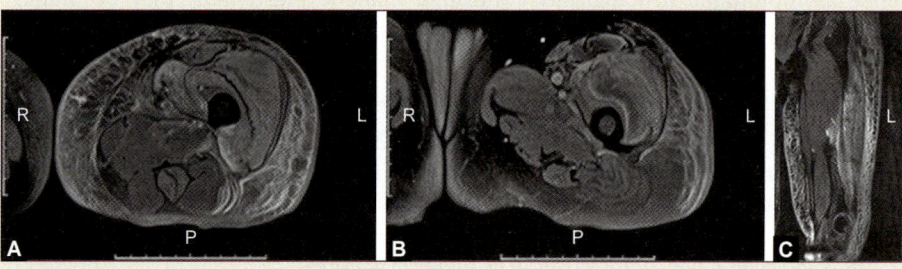

FIGS. 1A TO C: MRI of the left thigh of the patient.

DISCUSSION

Diabetic myonecrosis (DMN), also known as diabetic muscle infarction, is an under-recognized complication of poorly controlled long-standing diabetes mellitus. It was first described in 1965, and since then there has been well documented case reports and case series describing the same.

The mean duration of diabetes at the time of diagnosis is around 10–20 years, highlighting the fact that DMN is usually seen in patients with advanced diabetes. Nephropathy is commonly seen in three quarters of DMN, while half of the patients have concurrent retinopathy, neuropathy and nephropathy. Certainly most patients are initially misdiagnosed as cellulitis, and in many occasions, would have received prolonged courses of antibiotics before a final diagnosis is made.

Diabetic myonecrosis should be suspected in patients with long-standing diabetes presenting with acute muscular pain and swelling. There is usually no history of trauma and about 90% of patients are afebrile on admission. Routine laboratory tests usually do not aid in pinpointing the diagnosis. White blood cell count (WBC), erythrocyte sedimentation rate (ESR) and C-reactive protein (CRP) are usually elevated in 40%, 85% and 90% respectively. Creatinine kinase (CK) values are usually normal in 70% cases.

Radiological evaluation by ultrasound may help exclude pus collection but MRI remains the modality of choice. T2-weighted image reveal a hyperintense signal, while the T1-weighted image show an isotense to hypotense signal with associated perifascial, perimuscular, or subcutaneous edema.

Although muscle biopsy provides a definite diagnosis, it is not routinely recommended as it may unnecessarily delay the time to symptomatic improvement (almost double), apart from procedure related complications. Hence, muscle biopsy should only be reserved when the presentation is atypical and the diagnosis is unclear. Initial findings on biopsy reveals areas of muscle necrosis and edema. Subsequently fibrotic tissue and muscle fibre regeneration with lymphocytic infiltration is found.

DIFFERENTIAL DIAGNOSIS

The importance of DMN lies in the fact that it is underdiagnosed because the diagnosis is overlooked in favor of cellulitis and deep venous thrombosis. Table 1 below enumerates the various differential diagnosis and their clinical features.

TABLE 1: The differential diagnosis of DMN including clinical features and radiological appearances.

Disease condition	Major clinical features	Ultrasound findings	MRI findings
Diabetic myonecrosis	Tender, swollen muscle No overlying erythema	Nonspecific muscle edema No pus collection Sub- and interfascial fluid	T1: Subtle loss of intermuscular septae T2: Subcutaneous and intramuscular edema, sub- and interfascial fluid
Deep venous thrombosis	Tender, swollen muscle with overlying erythema	Clot in deep vein	
Cellulitis	Swollen extremity, raised temperature, tender, erythematous skin	Subcutaneous edema, extrafascial fluid	Subcutaneous edema and extrafascial fluid collection
Abscess	Swollen tender muscle increased temperature	Localized fluid collection	Peripherally enhancing fluid collection with extensive surrounding edema
Necrotizing fasciitis	Local tenderness and pain, swollen limb, systemic signs of infection (fever)	Muscle edema, subfascial fluid, limited by soft tissue air if present is suggestive	MRI—similar to DMN Contrast CT—soft tissue swelling + Heterogeneously enhancing muscles + Soft tissue air

(CT: computed tomography; DMN: diabetic myonecrosis; MRI: magnetic resonance imaging)

MANAGEMENT

There is no single intervention that shortens the recovery time and the existing treatment recommendations are based on limited evidence. The usual recommendation includes rest, analgesia and rigorous glycemic control. Low dose aspirin has been shown in some studies to reduce the recovery time. There is very limited data regarding anticoagulant use. Surgical intervention is not recommended as it may actually increase the recovery time.

Short-term recovery is usually excellent with most patients having complete resolution of symptoms in 4–6 weeks. However, it is important to remember that there is high 5-year mortality from underlying diabetes complications.

There is a high risk of recurrence occurring at the rate of about 35–45%. In one series, patients in whom NSAID (most commonly aspirin 81–325 mg/day were used) had the lowest recurrence.

Take Home Messages

- Diabetic myonecrosis is an underdiagnosed complication of diabetes mellitus
- Diabetic myonecrosis must be suspected in a long-standing poorly controlled diabetic presenting with acute muscle pain and limb swelling
- Rest, analgesia, good glycemic control and aspirin remain the mainstay of treatment
- Although there is good recovery, in the long term there is a high 5-year mortality from diabetes complications.

SUGGESTED READING

1. Gupta S, Goyal P, Sharma P, et al. Recurrent diabetic myonecrosis—an under-diagnosed cause of acute painful swollen limb in long-standing diabetics. Ann Med Surg. 2018;35:141-5.
2. Horton WB, Taylor JS, Ragland TJ, et al. Diabetic muscle infarction: a systematic review. BMJ Open Diabetes Research and Care. 2015;3:e000082.

CASE 8 | Heart Failure as a Presentation of Diabetes
Nilanjan Sengupta, Sajal Kamat

CASE HISTORY

A 53-year-old male businessman, who is obese and a foodie, nonsmoker and a social drinker, but not known to suffer from any chronic illness presented amidst the Durga Puja festivities with acute respiratory distress. ECG done at the time of presentation was unremarkable except for sinus tachycardia (Fig. 1). However, echocardiography demonstrated an ejection fraction (EF) of 18% with global hypokinesia (Fig. 2). As a part of routine metabolic workup, he was found to have diabetes with initial HbA1c of 15%, dyslipidemia and asymptomatic hyperuricemia. His renal function was normal. However,

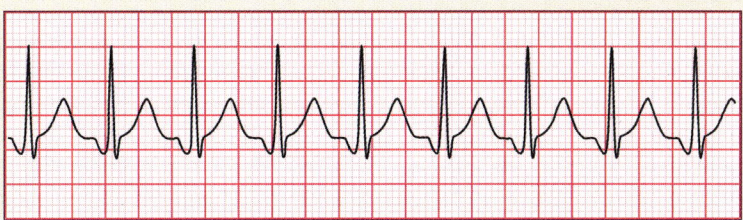

FIG. 1: Electrocardiogram (ECG) of the patient showing sinus tachycardia.

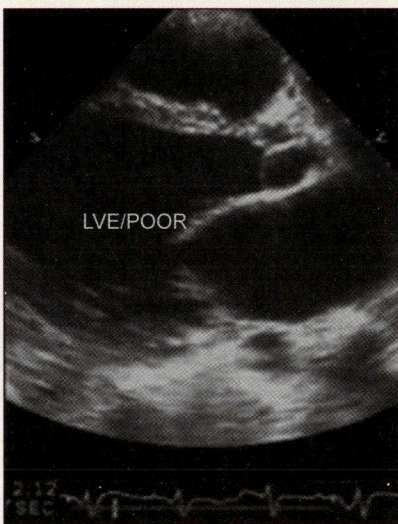

FIG. 2: 2D Echocardiography of the patient showing dilated ventricles with global hypokinesia.

the patient did not volunteer any osmotic symptoms, other symptoms attributable to diabetes or any effort angina or any other symptom attributable to coronary artery disease (CAD) prior to this presentation.

He was managed at hospital with standard antifailure therapy and glycemic control was achieved with multi-dose subcutaneous insulin (MSI) (regular insulin and glargine) and he was also put on empagliflozin, febuxostat and statin postdischarge by the endocrinologist. A coronary angiogram showed severe triple vessel disease with stenosis of >90% in the LAD. He was subsequently subjected to a planned coronary artery bypass grafting and put on lifestyle modification and guideline directed medical therapy for CAD along with. Subsequently, his glycemic control could be optimized with empagliflozin and metformin alone. He could undergo weight loss to the tune of 10 kg and there was a significant improvement in the cardiac function (EF-52%) and HbA1c (6.8%), 6 months following the initial presentation. He was completely asymptomatic at the time of the latest follow-up visits with the cardiologist and the endocrinologist.

INTRODUCTION

Diabetes and heart failure are closely related. Diabetes mellitus is highly prevalent among patients with heart failure, especially those with heart failure and preserved ejection fraction (HFpEF). Diabetic patients have an increased risk of developing heart failure because of the abnormal cardiac handling of glucose and free fatty acids. The prevalence of heart failure in diabetes is as high as 25% for chronic heart failure and up to 40% for acute heart failure. Its prevalence is four times higher in diabetics than that of general population. The common causes of heart failure in diabetes are CAD, ischemic cardiomyopathy and diabetic cardiomyopathy (due to microvascular dysfunction).

DISCUSSION

Type 2 diabetes mellitus (T2DM) is associated with a 4-fold increase in the risk of heart failure even after adjustment for other cardiovascular risk factors such as hypertension, cholesterol level, obesity and history of coronary artery disease. A number of structural, functional and metabolic factors in diabetes have been implicated in the increased risk of maladaptive remodelling that leads to heart failure, which is clinically manifested as serial wall motion changes, reduced regional ejection fraction, and increased end-diastolic and end-systolic volumes.

CONCLUSION

Atherosclerotic cardiovascular disease is a common companion of T2DM and an important factor for morbidity and mortality. Early recognition of diabetes and heart disease and their effective treatment can go a long way in reducing mortality and improving quality of life.

Take Home Messages

- *Both type 2 diabetes mellitus and heart failure can be quite advanced yet asymptomatic. In this case heart failure due to ASCVD was the presenting feature of T2DM*
- *In patients with cardiovascular comorbidities in diabetes, apart from guideline directed medical treatment and revascularization procedures as effective and applicable, right choice of antihyperglycemic agent is also very crucial. The current ADA-EASD hyperglycemia treatment algorithm is a useful and practical guide to approach such patients in clinical practice (Fig. 3)*
- *Whether urate lowering therapy in asymptomatic hyperuricemia does offer any cardiovascular benefit is still debatable but the patient was given the benefit of therapy in view of advanced atherosclerotic cardiovascular disease*
- *Empagliflozin was considered as an important agent for glycemic control in this patient from the very beginning except in the perioperative period in view of its benefits in heart failure and atherosclerotic cardiovascular disease*
- *The patient was also offered GLP-1 receptor agonist. However, he was not interested to start the same in view of the injectable nature of the drug and the fact that he could lose weight appreciably with therapeutic lifestyle change alone aided by empagliflozin.*

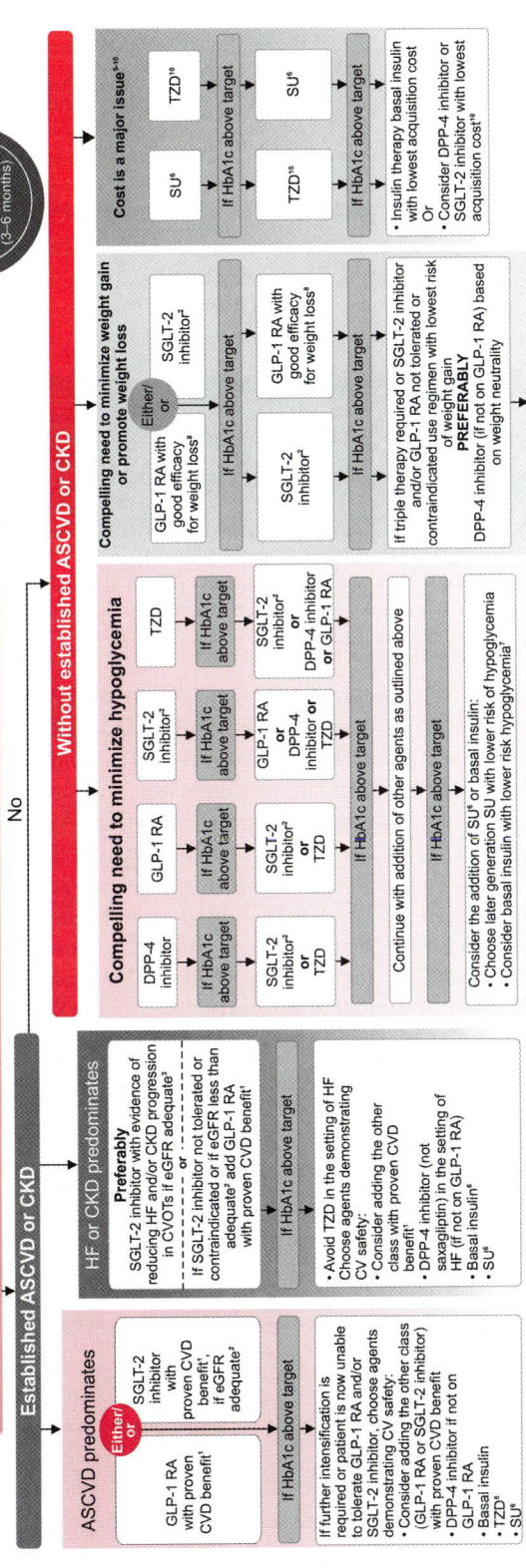

FIG. 3: ADA-EASD 2019 hyperglycemia treatment algorithm.
(ASCVD: atherosclerotic cardiovascular disease; CKD: chronic kidney disease; CV: cardiovascular; CVD: cardiovascular disease; DPP-4: dipeptidyl peptidase-4; eGFR: estimated glomerular filtration rate; GLP-1 RA: glucagon-like peptide-1 receptor agonist; HbA1c: glycosylated hemoglobin; HF: heart failure; SGLT-2: sodium-glucose cotransporter-2; SU: sulfonylurea; TZD: thiazolidinediones)

SUGGESTED READING

1. Brownlee M, Aiello L, Cooper M, Vinik A, Plutzky J, Boulton A. Williams Textbook of Endocrinology. Chapter 33, Complications of Diabetes Mellitus . 13th ed. Philadelphia: Elsevier/Saunders; c2016, Pages 1557-58.
2. Michael T, Nesto J, Nesto R. Joslin's Diabetes Mellitus. Chapter 58, Diabetes Mellitus and Heart Disease. 14th ed. Boston: Lippincott Williams and Wilkins; c2005.
3. Saely C, Vathie K, Drexel H. Holt Textbook of Diabetes. Chapter 41, Congestive Heart Failure. 5th ed. West Sussex: Wiley-Blackwell; c2007. Pages 684-97.

CASE 9: Antihyperglycemic Agents and Hospitalization for Heart Failure: A Practical Issue

Samit Ghosal

CASE HISTORY

A 53-year-old male nonsmoker business executive was being seen for the last 4 years. He had a 6-year history of type 2 diabetes mellitus (T2DM) controlled on metformin alone, 1.5 g/day and hypertension for 8 years controlled on amlodipine 5 mg/day. During his last visit 6 months ago, there was an elevated albumin creatinine ratio of 167 mg/g, but no other evidence of micro- or macrovascular complications. His HbA1c was 7.2%. This time the patient presented with increasing shortness of breath and fatigue. He said that he could not comfortably walk for more than 50 meters. On examination, he had bibasilar crackles and an elevated jugular venous pressure (JVP). His HbA1c now was 8.5%, low-density lipoprotein (LDL) cholesterol was 54 mg/dL, on atorvastatin and estimated glomerular filtration rate (eGFR) was calculated at over 60 mL/min.

As the patient looked quite unwell, hospitalization was advised. Chest X-ray showed cardiomegaly and small bilateral pleural effusions. ECG showed right bundle branch block (RBBB). NT-proB-type natriuretic peptide (BNP) was elevated at 215 pg/mL (normal up to 125 pg/mL). Echocardiogram showed a left ventricular ejection fraction (LVEF) of 54% with no regional wall motion abnormality and an E/A ratio of 1.2. There was no evidence of infection and liver function test (LFT) and thyroid functions were normal.

Amlodipine was changed to furosemide 20 mg twice daily. After some debate, empagliflozin 10 mg once daily was added.

The patient improved rapidly and his symptoms disappeared. He was sent home after 2 days.

DISCUSSION

- Heart failure is a complex clinical syndrome
- Typical symptoms and signs on exertion/rest
- Secondary to an abnormality of cardiac structure or function

- Impairs the ability of the heart to fill with blood at normal pressure or eject blood sufficient to fulfil the needs of the metabolizing organs
- Hospitalization due to heart failure: At least two of the following—Dyspnea, fatigue, ↓ exercise tolerance, other symptoms of volume overload.

At least two physical examination findings or one physical examination plus at least one laboratory finding: P/E (edema, ascites, basal crackles, ↑ JVP, S3 gallop, rapid weight gain), laboratory (NT-proBNP >2,000 pg/mL, radiological evidence of volume overload, Echo: E/e' >15, right heart).

Hospitalization for heart failure (hHF) can be a consequence of an established HF or a primary event. In this patient hHF was a primary event.

HOSPITALIZATION FOR HEART FAILURE EPIDEMIOLOGY BASICS

Incidence
- Rate ratio starts increasing significantly from 30 years of age irrespective of sex and keeps on increasing steeply beyond 80 years of age
- The rate ratio doubles in females with T2DM compared to their male counterpart once the age crosses 50 years
- 65% of these patients will have HFpEF (heart failure with preserved ejection fraction).

ASSOCIATED MORTALITY
- The hazard ratio (HR) for mortality after a single episode of hHF is 6-fold higher compared to a T2DM patient without a single admission for the same
- This mortality risk is highest within 0–1-month postdischarge from the hospital.

Risk Factors Predicting Hospitalization for Heart Failure
- Clinical identification: Age [>35 years (male) and >40 years (female)], past history of HF, past history of CAD, elevated blood urea and per 1% rise in HbA1c from baseline
- T2DM patients aged <55 years is at a high risk for hHF irrespective of the presence of albuminuria. However, the risk of hHF doubles from normo- to microalbuminuria. In contrast T2DM patient ≥75 years are at lower risk of hHF-I when they are normo-albuminuric. The risk starts increasing with albuminuria.

Risk Factors Identified for this Patient
- Age: 53 years
- Glycosylated hemoglobin: 8.5%
- Urine albumin creatinine ratio: 167 mg/g
- Breathlessness on effort.

SCREENING FOR HOSPITALIZATION FOR HEART FAILURE
- NT-ProBNP: >125 pg/mL needs further evaluation (ESC 2016, NICE 2018).

Issues Related to Use of NT-ProB-type Natriuretic Peptide
- High specificity with low sensitivity. That is the test helps ruling out heart failure pretty convincingly but can poorly make a confirmatory diagnosis
- Clinical conditions which can affect NT-ProBNP assay are shown in Table 1.

TABLE 1: Factors affecting the BNP assay.

Reduced levels of NT-ProBNP	Elevated levels of NT-ProBNP
• Afro-Caribbean origin • Treatment with diuretics, angiotensin-converting enzyme inhibitor, angiotensin receptor blockers, mineralocorticoid receptor antagonists, β-blockers	• Age >70 years • Left ventricular hypertrophy • Right ventricle overload • Tachycardia • Pulmonary embolism • Estimated glomerular filtration rate <60 mL/min • Sepsis • Chronic obstructive pulmonary disease • Cirrhosis of liver
There were no confounding factors in the patient under discussion.	

CONFIRMING DIAGNOSIS: ECHOCARDIOGRAPHY

Options
a. Refer the patient to cardiologist for further care
b. Carry on all by yourself as far as it is possible.

Going Ahead with Option (b)
Remember to request for the E/A and E/e' ratio while requesting for an echocardiography. Parameters of the patient under discussion:
- NT-ProBNP: 215 pg/mL
- Echocardiography basics:
    - LVEF: 54% (no regional wall motion abnormalities or LVH)
    - E/A ratio 1.2.

MANAGEMENT ISSUES

General Management
- Rule out liver dysfunction, hypothyroidism and infection.

Specific Management

TABLE 2: Factors concerning survival, symptoms and prevention of heart failure.

Survival	Symptoms	Preventing hHF
• Loop diuretics (Class II B-CHAMPION trial) • Mineralocorticoid receptor antagonist (Class II A-TOPCAT trial)	• Isosorbide mononitrate: Class III—NEAT-HFpEF trial)	• SGLT-2 inhibitor: (EMPA-REG, CANVAS Program and DECLARE-TIMI 58)

(hHF: hospitalization for heart failure)

- E/A ratio >1: Diuretic (TOPCAT trial): Target to bring down the ratio <1
- E/A ratio 0.8–1.0: Ivabradine to reduce heart rate (SWEDIC trial).

> **Take Home Messages**
> - *Preventing hHF: Add a SGLT-2 inhibitor ± other medications as required to get to glycemic target without increasing hHF risk*
> - *Substitute CCB with diuretics or add a diuretic*
> - *Adding a SGLT2 inhibitor to a loop diuretic will increase diuresis and may cause problems. However, in this patient, it was decided to do so. The patient was informed that he would have polyuria.*

SUGGESTED READING

1. Heart Foundation. (2018). Heart Failure Guidelines 2018: Key Messages and Frequently asked questions. [online] Available from https://www.heartfoundation.org.au/images/uploads/publications/HF_Key_Messages_and_FAQs.pdf [Last accessed June, 2019].
2. McAllister DA, Read SH, Kerssens J, et al. Incidence of Hospitalization for Heart Failure and Case-Fatality Among 3.25 Million People With and Without Diabetes Mellitus. Circulation. 2018;138:2774-86.
3. Mitter SS, Shah SJ, Thomas JD. A Test in Context: E/A and E/e' to Assess Diastolic Dysfunction and LV Filling Pressure. J Am Coll Cardiol. 2017;69(11):1451-64.
4. National Institute for Health and Care Excellence. (2018). Chronic heart failure in adults: diagnosis and management. NICE guideline. [online] Available from https://www.nice.org.uk/guidance/ng106 [Last accessed June, 2019].
5. Neal B, Perkovic V, Mahaffey KW, et al. Canagliflozin and Cardiovascular and Renal Events in Type 2 Diabetes. N Engl J Med. 2017;377:644-57.
6. Ponikowsky P, Voors AA, Anker SD, et al. 2016 ESC Guidelines for the diagnosis and treatment of acute and chronic heart failure: The Task Force for the diagnosis and treatment of acute and chronic heart failure of the European Society of Cardiology (ESC) Developed with the special contribution of the Heart Failure Association (HFA) of the ESC. Eur Heart J. 2016;37:2129-200.
7. Rosengren A, Edqvist J, Rawshani A, et al. Excess risk of hospitalisation for heart failure among people with type 2 diabetes. Diabetologia. 2018;61:2300-9.
8. Sabatasso S, Vaucher P, Augsburger M, et al. Sensitivity and specificity of NT-proBNP to detect heart failure at post mortem examination. Int J Legal Med. 2011;125(6):849-56.
9. Savarese G, Lund LH. Global Public health burden of heart failure. Card Fail Rev. 2017;3(1):7-11.
10. Solomon SD, Dobson J, Pocock S, et al. Influence of Nonfatal Hospitalization for Heart Failure on Subsequent Mortality in Patients With Chronic Heart Failure. Circulation. 2007;116:1482-7.
11. Williams B, Gandhi P. A Risk Prediction Model for Heart Failure Hospitalization among Patients with Type 2 Diabetes. Diabetes. 2018;67(Suppl 1). [online] Available from https://doi.org/10.2337/db18-409-P [Last accessed June, 2019].
12. Wiviott SD, Raz I, Bonaca MP, et al. Dapagliflozin and Cardiovascular Outcomes in Type 2 Diabetes. N Engl J Med. 2019;380:347-57.
13. Zakeri R, Cowie MR. Heart failure with preserved ejection fraction: controversies, challenges and future directions. Heart. 2018;104:377-84.
14. Zinman B, Wanner C, Lachin JM, et al. Empagliflozin, Cardiovascular Outcomes, and Mortality in Type 2 Diabetes. N Engl J Med. 2015;373:2117-28.

CASE 10
Modern Management of Type 2 Diabetes Mellitus: Making Sense of the Multiple Options

Samit Ghosal

CASE HISTORY

A 56-year-old school teacher, had type 2 diabetes mellitus (T2DM) for the last 2 years, and managed on metformin 1.5 g/day. He has a history of hypertension for the last 6 years and managed on losartan-hydrochlorothiazide combination. His BMI is 30, HbA1c is 8.1% and BP is 145/86 mm Hg. Peripheral pulses are normal and the fundi are clear. His eGFR is over 60 mL/min. Dapagliflozin 5 mg before breakfast was added to his regimen. Six months later his HbA1c was 7.1%.

DISCUSSION

Defining the term "Management of T2DM": *WHO Standards of Care and Clinical Practice Guidelines*:

WHO recommendations
- Relieving symptoms
- Correcting associated health problems and reduce morbidity, mortality and economic costs of diabetes
- Preventing as much as possible acute and long-term complications; monitoring the development of complications and providing timely intervention
- Improving quality of life and productivity of the individual with diabetes.

All diabetes-related recommendations jettisoned the glucocentric approach as early as the early 90s. It is a futile strategy which lowers glucose without having an impact on the extremely morbid outcomes associated with it. This is reflected in the present-day global disease burden and future projections recently published in *The Lancet* with the combination of myocardial infarction and stroke accounting for nearly 80% of mortality.

Today we can make a difference in outcomes using the modern management tools at our disposal. With the plethora of agents available, the question is how?
The management issues in this patient are simple but require some thought.

Achieving glycosylated hemoglobin (HbA1c) target. What is the target?
Achieving HbA1c target: There are a couple of important practical considerations before approaching this issue:

What is the HbA1c target?	<ul><li><7.0% (American Diabetes Association)</li><li><6.5% (American Association of Clinical Endocrinologists)</li><li>7.0–8.0% (American College of Physicians)</li></ul>
How do we achieve this target?	<ul><li>Without inducing hypoglycemia and/or weight gain</li><li>Stepwise versus combination approach</li></ul>

What is the HbA1c target?

The target HbA1c is not based on the idea of reducing glucose per se, but translation of that value/range into outcomes benefit. When we talk about outcomes there are two broad classifications for the same—microvascular (nephropathy, retinopathy and neuropathy) and macrovascular (CV disease, stroke and peripheral vascular disease).

TABLE 1: Median glycosylated hemoglobin (HbA1c) achieved in various studies.

Studies	UKPDS 33	UKPDS—10-year follow-up	ACCORD	ADVANCE
Median HbA1c achieved (%)	7.0	8.1	6.3	6.5
Outcomes benefit	Microvascular	• Microvascular • Coronary events • All-cause mortality	Mixed bag	Microvascular

As we can see from most of the trials done comparing intensive versus conventional diabetes management strategies, there is no additional advantage going below an HbA1c of 7.0%.
- The legacy effect of early effective glucose control as suggested by UKPDS also supports an HbA1c range of 7.0–8.0%
- Recent CVOTs with flozins, for example, had to document glycemic equipoise prior to drawing any form of conclusions. In all these studies the end-of-trial HbA1c was above 7.0%.

Hence, from a practical point of view an HbA1c target of 7.0–7.5% seems reasonable.

How do we achieve this target?

Having set our glycemic target, it is extremely important to formulate an effective strategy to achieve our aim.

Broad strategy: Achieving HbA1c target without inducing hypoglycemia and/or weight gain. Any form of hypoglycemia severely compromises the quality of life and the sense of ill-being can persist for an entire day. However, the scare of adverse cardiac and cerebrovascular outcomes is exclusively associated with severe hypoglycemia, which needs to be avoided at all cost. This is of prime consideration in the elderly.

The issue of weight should also be considered in perspective. To make a difference in outcomes we need at least a 10% reduction in weight from baseline, which none of the available anti-hyperglycemics are capable of providing at the present time.

Specific strategy: A couple of head-to-head randomized controlled trials have confirmed the superiority of the aggressive combination therapy approach compared to the traditional stepwise approach as far as achieving and maintaining the target HbA1c is concerned.

TABLE 2: List of recent combination medication studies.

Trial	Combination agents used
EDICT	Metformin + Pioglitazone + GLP1-RA + Basal insulin
QATAR	Metformin + SU + Pioglitazone + GLP1-RA

Advantages of such a strategy:
- Early achievement of metabolic target
- Long-term durability
- De-escalation as required
- Lower risk of hypoglycemia and glycemic variability versus staggered traditional approach.

Research recommendation:
- Outcomes benefit is not fully established.

We can improvize and prepare our own combination based on patient's baseline HbA1c, other metabolic parameters, weight, propensity to hypoglycemia, associated comorbidities, etc.

Preventing complications: How?
- Achieving HbA1c and other metabolic targets
- Choosing drugs capable of doing so in preference to those which cannot.

There are today few molecules within three drug classes capable of altering diabetes-related outcomes:
1. Gliptins in CARMELINA have reduced new onset or progressive retinopathy and new onset or persistent macroalbuminuria
2. Flozins in EMPAREG, CREDENCE, CANVAS and DECLARE-Timi 58 have reduced ESRD, renal death CV death and hospitalization due to heart failure
3. Glucagon like peptide 1 receptor agonists (GLP-1 RAs) in LEADER, HARMONY, REWIND, SUSTAIN-6 have reduced MI, nonfatal stroke and acute coronary mortality.

Take Home Messages

How do we implement evidence-based management strategy to the patient under discussion?
Step 1: Initiate agents which can alter outcomes
Step 2: Complement with agents aiding in achieving HbA1c target
Step 3: Tackle other comorbidities aggressively

1. Stepwise approach:
- *Ideal scenario: SGLT-2i or GLP1-RA (with proven outcomes benefit)*
- *Cost constraint: SGLT-2i or pioglitazone (trade off: weight gain)*
- *Severe cost constraint: Pioglitazone or SU (glimeperide or gliclazide, with proven CV safety).*

2. Combination therapy:
- *Ideal scenario: SGLT-2i and GLP1-RA (with proven outcomes benefit)*
- *Not willing for early injectable initiation: SGLT-2i and Gliptin*
- *Cost constraints: Pioglitazone and SGLT-2i*
- *Severe cost constraint: Pioglitazone and SU (with proven CV safety).*

SUGGESTED READING

1. Abdul-Ghani MA, Migahid O, Megahed A, et al. Combination Therapy With Exenatide Plus Pioglitazone Versus Basal/Bolus Insulin in Patients With Poorly Controlled Type 2 Diabetes on Sulfonylurea Plus Metformin: The Qatar Study. Diabetes Care. 2017;40:325-31.
2. Abdul-Ghani MA, Puckett C, Triplett C, et al. Initial combination therapy with metformin, pioglitazone and exenatide is more effective than sequential add-on therapy in subjects with new-onset diabetes. Results from the Efficacy and Durability of Initial Combination Therapy for Type 2 Diabetes (EDICT): a randomized trial. Diabetes Obes Metab. 2015;17:268-75.
3. American Diabetes Association. Glycemic Targets: Standards of Medical Care in Diabetes—2018. Diabetes Care. 2018;41:S55-64.
4. Garber AJ, Abrahamson MJ, Barzilay JI, et al. Consensus statement by the American association of clinical endocrinologists and American college of endocrinology on the comprehensive Type 2 diabetes management algorithm—2018 executive summary. Endocr Pract. 2018;24:91-120.
5. GBD 2016 Causes of Death Collaborators. Global, regional, and national age-sex specific mortality for 264 causes of death, 1980–2016: a systematic analysis for the Global Burden of Disease Study 2016. Lancet. 2017;390:1151-210.

6. Gerstein HC, Miller ME, Byington RP, et al. Effects of intensive glucose lowering in Type 2 diabetes. N Engl J Med. 2008;358:2545-59.
7. Patel A, MacMahon S, Chalmers J, et al. Intensive blood glucose control and vascular outcomes in patients with Type 2 diabetes. N Engl J Med. 2008;358:2560-72.
8. Qaseem A, Wilt TJ, Kansagara D, et al. Hemoglobin A1c targets for glycemic control with pharmacologic therapy for nonpregnant adults with Type 2 diabetes mellitus: a guidance statement update from the American college of physicians. Ann Intern Med. 2018;168:569-76.
9. UK Prospective Diabetes Study (UKPDS) Group. Effect of intensive blood-glucose control with metformin on complications in overweight patients with Type 2 diabetes (UKPDS 34). Lancet. 1998;352:854-65.
10. WHO. (1994). Management of diabetes mellitus Standards of care and Clinical Practice Guidelines. [online] Available from http://applications.emro.who.int/dsaf/dsa509.pdf [Last accessed June, 2019].

CASE 11: Approach to a Patient of Type 2 Diabetes Mellitus with Unexplained Hyperglycemic State

Sanjay Chatterjee

CASE HISTORY

A patient with long-standing type 2 diabetes mellitus (T2DM) and comorbidities.

A 68-year-old female observed sudden increase in her blood glucose values over the last 6 weeks. She lived with her husband. She had one daughter who lived in the United Kingdom. She is a nonsmoker and is a social drinker. She was diagnosed with T2DM in the year 1998 and was treated with metformin along with lifestyle management. She was told about the beneficial effects of blood glucose control and she was always adherent to her diet, exercise and medication quite rigorously. At the time of her consultation in July 2016, she was taking sitagliptin 100 mg, metformin 1,000 mg, injection glargine 10–14 units [depending on her fasting capillary blood glucose (CBG) levels], telmisartan 40 mg and rosuvastatin 10 mg daily.

Till the end of May 2016, her self-monitored CBG levels were: fasting 95–120 mg/dL, postmeal values between 130 mg/dL and 160 mg/dL. Her last HbA1c value measured in May 2016 was 6.8%.

Her recent CBG values since June 2016 were: fasting 150–200 mg/dL; postmeal values were between 190 mg/dL and 260 mg/dL.

Laboratory results (July 2016) showed:
- Hemoglobin: 12.8 g/dL; white blood cells: 8,800/mm^3
- FPG: 208 mg/dL; postbreakfast plasma glucose: 258 mg/dL; HbA1c: 8.2%
- Creatinine: 0.9 mg/dL; SGPT: 36 U/L; SGOT: 33 U/L
- Serum cholesterol: 166 mg/dL; triglyceride: 214 mg/dL
- HDL-cholesterol: 36 mg/dL; LDL-cholesterol: 99 mg/dL
- Thyroid-stimulating hormone: 3.2 µIU/mL; Uric acid: 6.6 mg/dL
- Urine routine examination showed presence of glucose +
- Urine culture was sterile.

While taking her history of concomitant medication, it was known that in the first week of June 2016, she consulted an orthopedic surgeon for her aches and pains in left knee, aggravated by climbing of stairs. Her orthopedic surgeon prescribed her glucosamine sulfate along with other medicines.

She was asked to stop glucosamine sulfate and to talk to her orthopedic surgeon about alternate medications. Antihyperglycemic medications were unaltered. After 1 month, when she came for follow-up, her FPG was 123 mg/dL; and PPG was 160 mg/dL. Her self-monitored blood glucose values were similar.

DISCUSSION (TABLE 1)

Since the time of publication of UKPDS study, management of T2DM took a new turn and the outlook of diabetes management changed dramatically. Prior to UKPDS, there was no evidence that glycemic control could prevent development and progression of diabetic complications. The results of the UKPDS unequivocally proved the benefit of control of blood glucose. It was further seen that beyond a threshold value of HbA1c 7%, diabetic complications start emerging. Since then, the physicians around the world took great interest in control of blood glucose and patients, particularly the educated ones, followed the same.

Researchers in the field of diabetes also wanted to see whether the benefit increased in targeting to achieve an HbA1c level of 6.5% or, even 6% in (i) well-controlled patients, (ii) poorly controlled patients and (iii) patients with cardiovascular comorbidities. Although the results in the first group were satisfactory but same was not observed in other groups or, rather proved to be detrimental to patients.

TABLE 1: Drugs that increase blood glucose.

Drug that increase blood glucose	Mechanism	Incidence of hyperglycemia (%)	Reversibility
Androgen deprivation therapy	Increased insulin resistance	20–30%	Yes
Somatostatin analogs	Inhibition of insulin secretion	30%	Yes
Glucocorticoids	Decreased insulin secretion and increased gluconeogenesis	65%	Yes
mTOR inhibitors/immuno-suppressive agent	Decreased insulin secretion and action	10–50%	Yes
Tyrosine kinase inhibitors	Insulin resistance	20–36%	Yes
Thiazide diuretics	Decreased insulin secretion and sensitivity	11%	Yes
Statins	Decreased insulin secretion and action	9–12%	Yes
Antipsychotics	Decreased insulin secretion and action due to antagonism at peripheral muscarinic receptors	22%	Yes
Antiretroviral therapy	Lipodystrophy, insulin resistance and mitochondrial dysfunction	0.5%	No
Interferon-α	Immunological beta cell destruction	0.34%	No

The recent consensus among physicians across the world is to achieve glycemic target on an individualized basis rather than targeting to achieve HbA1c of 7% or, less, irrespective of age or comorbidities.

Glucosamine is a hexosamine and is present in synovial fluids as lubricant. In many patients with T2DM it abruptly increases insulin resistance and worsens glycemic control. Glucosamine is a widely used dietary supplement that is described as efficacious and safe for many individuals with osteoarthritis, especially of the knees. Concerns that glucosamine consumption may worsen glucose tolerance and induce insulin resistance were based on small case reports (but not on any large-scale clinical observations) and on in vitro studies by Marshall et al., showing that exogenous glucosamine could increase the activity of the hexosamine biosynthesis pathway, a metabolic process that is believed to function as a nutrient sensor modulating insulin sensitivity and glucose uptake in peripheral tissues. The end-product of this pathway is UDP-N-acetylGlcN, a substrate for O-GlcNAc transferase, which mediates the addition of β-N-acetylGlcN to the hydroxyl groups of serine and/or threonine residues on a wide variety of proteins. This post-translational modification regulates a wide range of biological processes, including signal transduction/metabolic proteins that modulate glucose metabolism and insulin sensitivity. As reviewed by Copeland et al., there are strong associations between elevated GlcN acylation of proteins with glucose toxicity and impaired insulin signaling; excessive flux of sugars through the hexosamine signaling pathway has therefore been implicated as a causative factor in the development of T2DM or, worsening glycemia.

> ### Take Home Message
> - *The objective of this case presentation is to remind physicians and diabetologist of the facts that while dealing with a situation of sudden rise of blood glucose in an otherwise well-controlled patient with T2DM, history taking, particularly history of recent change in concomitant medication, is very important. Glucosamine-induced hyperglycemia is not very common, but it is worth remembering.*

SUGGESTED READING

1. American Diabetes Association. ADA Standards of Medical Care in Diabetes—2018. Diabetes Care. 2018;41(Suppl 1):S1-152.
2. Biggee BA, Blinn CM, Nuite M, et al. Effects of oral glucosamine sulphate on serum glucose and insulin during an oral glucose tolerance test of subjects with osteoarthritis. Ann Rheum Dis. 2007; 66(2):260-2.
3. Copeland RJ, Bullen JW, Hart GW. Cross-talk between GlcNAcylation and phosphorylation: roles in insulin resistance and glucose toxicity. Am J Physiol Endocrinol Metab. 2008;295:E17-28.
4. King P, Peacock I, Donnelly R. The UK prospective diabetes study (UKPDS): clinical and therapeutic implications for type 2 diabetes. Br J Clin Pharmacol. 1999;48(5):643-8.
5. Marshall S, Bacote V, Traxinger R. Discovery of a metabolic pathway mediating glucose-induced desensitization of the glucose transport system. Role of hexosamine biosynthesis in the induction of insulin resistance. J Biol Chem. 1991;266:4706-12.
6. Riddle MC. Effects of intensive glucose lowering in the management of patients with type 2 diabetes mellitus in the Action to Control Cardiovascular Risk in Diabetes (ACCORD) trial. Circulation. 2010;24;122(8):844-6.

CASE 12: Fibrocalculus Pancreatic Diabetes Presenting as Pancreatic Adenocarcinoma

Satinath Mukhopadhyay, Partha Pratim Chakraborty

CASE HISTORY

A 35-year-old man with diabetes for 11 years presented to our clinic with anorexia, loss of 10% of body weight in last 6 months and poor glycemic control for preceding 3 months. He initially responded to oral hypoglycemic drugs but had to be switched to twice daily premixed insulin 2 years back due to uncontrolled blood glucose. He did well with his prescribed insulin regimen until recently when he noticed persistent, uncontrolled hyperglycemia despite adhering to therapy. There was no history of ketoacidosis. Examination was significant for low body mass index (BMI) 16.9 kg/m^2, pallor, jaundice and no acanthosis. Baseline biochemistry is summarized in Table 1.

Ultrasonography of the upper abdomen revealed distended GB, chronic calcific pancreatitis with a mass in the head of the pancreas. Common bile duct (CBD) was distended (14 mm in diameter) and sludge with echoreflective foci was noted. A 3D CT scan of the abdomen showed bulky pancreatic head and neck with atrophy of the rest of the pancreas. The main pancreatic duct was dilated (7 mm) with multiple intraductal calculi in along its entire length (Figs. 1 and 2).

Magnetic resonance cholangiopancreatography (MRCP) showed dilated CBD (20 mm) with dilatation of the proximal intrahepatic and extrahepatic biliary tree (Fig. 3). Serum CA19-9 was elevated (630.38 U/L; normal <37). A diagnosis of pancreatic adenocarcinoma in the background of fibrocalculus pancreatic diabetes (FCPD) was made.

TABLE 1: Baseline biochemistry.

Test	Value
Hemoglobin	6.4 g/dL
Total leukocyte count	17,800/mm^3
Erythrocyte sedimentation rate	112 mm 1st hour
Total bilirubin	9.36 mg/dL
Direct	6.52 mg/dL
Indirect	2.84 mg/dL
Serum glutamic-oxaloacetic transaminase	87 U/L
Serum glutamic-pyruvic transaminase	126 U/L
Alkaline phosphatase	1,467 U/L
Total protein	6.8 g/dL
Albumin	3.2 g/dL
Globulin	3.6 g/dL

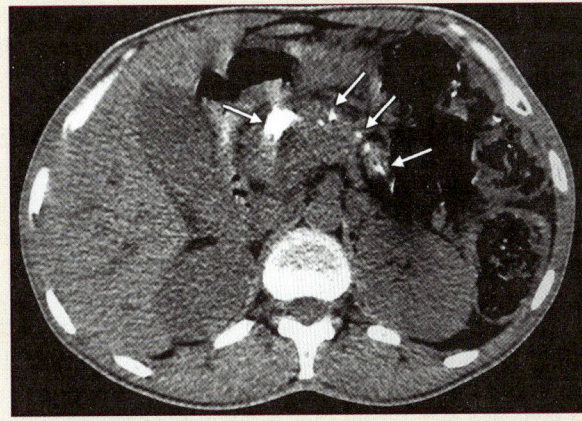

FIG. 1: CT scan of the abdomen showing calcifications over head, body, and tail of pancreas (white arrows) along the course of main pancreatic duct.

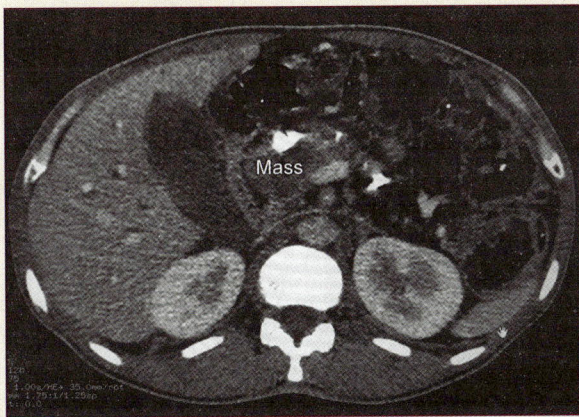

FIG. 2: Contrast-enhanced computed tomography (CECT) abdomen showing hypodense "mass" involving the head of pancreas.

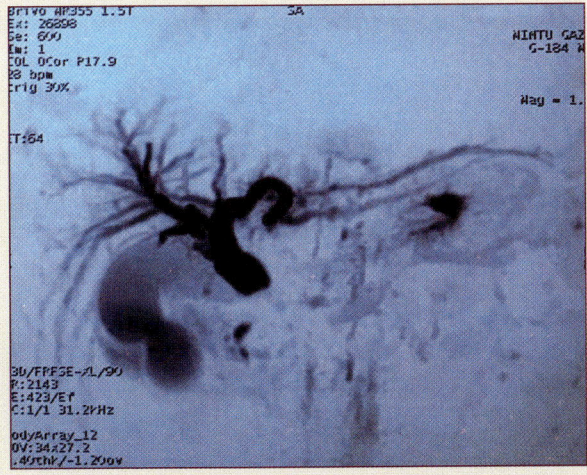

FIG. 3: Magnetic resonance cholangiopancreatography (MRCP) showing dilatation of common bile duct (CBD).

DISCUSSION

Tropical calcific pancreatitis (TCP) is a unique form of chronic pancreatitis of uncertain etiology, usually presenting with the classical features of pain abdomen and steatorrhea in childhood or adolescence, with evidence of pancreatic calculi along with atrophic pancreas on imaging. The condition is found predominantly in tropical and subtropical countries with the highest prevalence in the Indian states of Tamil Nadu and Kerala. When associated with diabetes, representing a more advanced stage of the disease, it is known as FCPD. FCPD constitutes <1% of all cases of diabetes. The risk of developing pancreatic cancer is the highest in patients with FCPD as compared to all other forms of pancreatitis and is believed to be 100-fold greater than those without FCPD. Pancreatic adenocarcinoma is the fourth most common cause of cancer death worldwide with extremely poor prognosis (5-year survival <3%). Association of diabetes with pancreatic cancer is bidirectional. While patients with diabetes have a 2-fold increase in the risk of pancreatic cancer, hyperglycemia may also result from the secretion of adrenomedullin or S-100 by pancreatic duct adenocarcinoma. Anorexia, pain abdomen and progressive weight loss are common presenting features with/without obstructive jaundice. Venous thrombosis, superficial or deep may be seen in some patients. Most FCPD patients with pancreatic adenocarcinoma experience worsening glycemic control before presentation.

> **Take Home Messages**
>
> - *Fibrocalcific pancreatic diabetes, a secondary form of diabetes, is not uncommon in India. It should be suspected in young, lean individuals with insulin requiring diabetes presenting with/without abdominal pain and/or steatorrhea. Presence of intraductal calculi with dilatation of the pancreatic duct is characteristic. Fecal chymotrypsin is a sensitive marker for FCPD. Association with SPINK gene polymorphism has been recently reported*
> - *Anorexia, weight loss and worsening glycemic control in a patient of FCPD should be treated as a warning signal for the treating physician and the patient should be evaluated for any occult pancreatic malignancy, even in the absence of classical signs of pancreatic cancer like obstructive jaundice, palpable gall bladder and pain abdomen*
> - *Since patients with FCPD have the highest risk of pancreatic cancer among all forms of pancreatitis, (absolute risk >100-fold), routine screening of all patients of FCPD with annual ultrasonography and serum CA19-9 may be of help in early detection pancreatic cancer in patients with FCPD.*

SUGGESTED READING

1. Barman KK, Premalatha G, Mohan V. Tropical chronic pancreatitis. Postgrad Med J. 2003;79:606-15.
2. Chakraborty PP, Dutta D, Biswas K, et al. Pancreatic carcinoma in fibrocalcific pancreatic diabetes: An eastern India perspective. Indian J Endocr Metab. 2012;16:S486-8.
3. Unnikrishnan R, Mohan V. Pancreatic diseases and diabetes. In: RIG H, Cockram C, Flyvbjerg A, Goldstein BJ, editors. Textbook of Diabetes. Vol. 18: Wiley Blackwell; 2004. p. 302.

CASE 13: Myonecrosis: An Unusual Microvascular Complication of Diabetes

Satinath Mukhopadhyay, Partha Pratim Chakraborty

CASE HISTORY

A 62-year-old lady with a 22-year history of type 2 diabetes mellitus (T2DM) presented with pain and swelling involving the anterior aspect of her right thigh for the preceding 10 days. The pain was of acute onset, constant and dull aching in nature and aggravated on movement of the involved leg. She denied any history of trauma, skin infection or administration of injection over the affected part. She was afebrile and could recall no similar illness in the past. The patient however noticed pain and numbness of both her feet for the last 2 years. She had been shifted to twice daily premixed insulin 6 months prior to her presentation to our clinic, due to failure to achieve glycemic control with oral antidiabetic agents. Her hypertension, detected 5 years back, was well-controlled with telmisartan 40 mg/day and hydrochlorothiazide 6.25 mg/day.

Clinical examination revealed the following:
Height: 157 cm, weight: 55 kg, body mass index (BMI): 22.3 kg/m^2, waist circumference: 93 cm. BP was 124/76 mm of Hg without significant postural drop. Knee jerks were diminished bilaterally; ankle jerks were absent. 10 g monofilament test: 3/6 bilaterally. Fundoscopy showed moderate nonproliferative diabetic retinopathy without clinically significant macular edema.

The girth of the right thigh was 52.5 cm and left thigh was 50 cm (Fig. 1). Although the anterior aspect of the right thigh was tender, the temperature difference between the two thighs was less than 2°C on infrared thermometry. The relevant investigations have been summarized in Table 1.

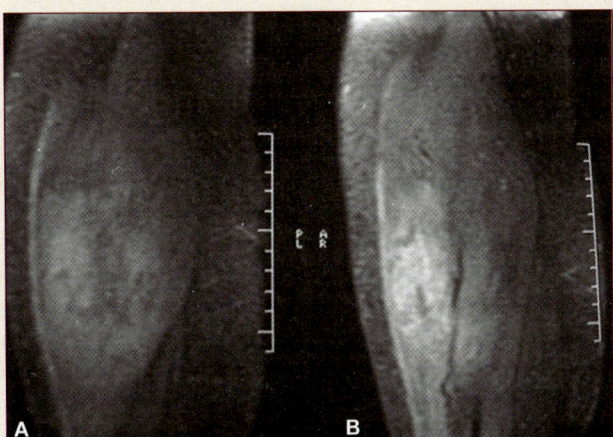

FIG. 1: (A) Increased swelling of the anterior aspect of the right thigh; (B) Increased signal intensity in STIR sequences on the lower half of the right vastus anterior muscle.

TABLE 1: Summary of investigations.

Parameters	Patient's value (Normal range)
Total leukocyte count	8,900/mm^3
Erythrocyte sedimentation rate	63 mm in first hour
Fasting plasma glucose	327 mg/dL
Postprandial plasma glucose	417 mg/dL
Creatine phosphokinase	311 U/L (<167)
Albumin/creatinine ratio	286 µg/mg
Glycosylated hemoglobin	10.8%
Estimated glomerular filtration rate	61 mL/min
Serum sodium	138 mEq/L
Serum potassium	3.8 mEq/L

USG of the right thigh revealed an ill-defined hypoechoic area (25 cm × 15 cm) with multiple internal echogenic lines over anterolateral aspect of the right quadriceps. No features of DVT were noted in the color Doppler study.

MRI of the right thigh: No significant alteration in signal intensity in T1-weighted image but diffusely increased signal intensity of subcutaneous fat, fascia and muscle was noted in T2-weighted images. Short tau inversion recovery (STIR) sequence revealed characteristic hyperintense signals involving vastus anterior in its lower-half, consistent with myonecrosis.

She was treated with basal-bolus insulin therapy to achieve glycemic control. Pain was relieved with nonsteroidal anti-inflammatory drug (NSAID). The swelling reduced gradually and she was discharged after 3 weeks with minimal swelling of the right thigh.

DISCUSSION

Diabetic myonecrosis is an uncommon complication of long-standing diabetes (average duration ~15 years). There is an increased predilection for females (F:M = 1.3–1.7:1) and type 1 diabetes mellitus (T1DM). Majority of such patients are in their 3rd or 4th decades of life and have coexistent microvascular complications (97%) either nephropathy (70%) or retinopathy (55%) or neuropathy (55%). Signs and symptoms of myonecrosis include abrupt onset of pain (80%), swelling of affected part (75.9%), palpable mass (33.7%) and fever (10.7%). Thigh muscles are most frequently involved (83.7%) followed by the calf muscles (19.3%). Bilateral involvement is seen in 8.4% of cases and upper limb involvement is extremely uncommon. Among the thigh muscles, quadriceps (vastus lateralis: 24%; vastus medialis: 22%) are involved in the majority.

The pathophysiology is yet unknown but arteriosclerosis and diabetic microangiopathy are the most plausible causes. Altered coagulation may also play a role. The disease is characterized by elevated ESR, CRP and CPK in half of the affected patients. Leukocytosis is seen only in about 8–14% of cases.

Diagnosis is confirmed by imaging the affected part. USG is characterized by well-marginated, hypoechoic, intramuscular lesion with internal linear echogenicities, as in this case. Lack of a predominantly anechoic area and absence of swirling/motion of fluid with pressure are typical sonological findings.

The CT appearances are diffuse muscular enlargement with decreased attenuation of the affected muscle (24 HU) and increased attenuation of the subcutaneous fat along with thickening of subcutaneous fascial planes and of the overlying skin. MRI is the imaging modality of choice that documents isointense or hypointense areas on T1-weighted images, secondary to increased water content from edema and inflammatory changes and increased signal intensity in T2-weighted images, STIR sequence and gadolinium-enhanced images. The other suggestive findings are diffuse enlargement with ill-defined borders secondary to loss of the normal fatty intramuscular septa and tiny foci of hyperintense signal consistent with foci of hemorrhages. Postcontrast study shows high signal intensity and small focal areas of rim enhancement that represent infarction or necrosis within the areas of ischemic muscle.

The list of differentials includes cellulitis, deep venous thrombosis, muscle abscess, tropical pyomyositis, thrombophlebitis, necrotising fasciitis, diabetic lumbosacral plexopathy, fracture/muscle rupture, hematoma. Typical findings observed in USG and MRI helps to reach a definitive diagnosis. Muscle biopsy should better be avoided as it may aggravate the condition.

Treatment includes bed rest and nonweight-bearing exercise, analgesia (narcotics, NSAIDs, icepacks) and glycemic control (reduced recurrence). Spontaneous recovery is seen in 4–8 weeks. However, recurrence is common (~50%) and usually involves a different muscle. Half of recurrences occur within 2 months and recurrence resolves rapidly. It carries a poor long-term prognosis as majority die within 5 years probably due to established vascular complications.

Take Home Messages

- *The differential diagnosis for unilateral pain and swelling of thigh in a patient with diabetes includes cellulitis, muscle abscess, tropical pyomyositis, thrombophlebitis, DVT, necrotizing fasciitis, diabetic lumbosacral plexopathy/diabetic amyotrophy, fracture/muscle rupture and hematoma*
- *Diabetic myonecrosis is an uncommon microvascular complication of diabetes. This is usually seen in long-standing diabetes, but may occur with short duration of disease. Other microvascular complications like nephropathy, neuropathy or retinopathy are usually present*
- *USG and MRI of the affected part are diagnostic for diabetic myonecrosis*
- *Avoid diagnostic muscle biopsy, as it may aggravate myonecrosis*
- *Symptomatic management is the cornerstone of therapy and there is no role of antibiotics.*

SUGGESTED READING

1. Gupta RD, Haobam SS, Krishna A, et al. Clinico-radiological characteristics and not laboratory markers are useful in diagnosing diabetic myonecrosis in Asian Indian patients with type 2 diabetes mellitus: A 10-year experience from South India. J Family Med Prim Care. 2018;7(6):1243-7.
2. Mazoch MJ, Bajaj G, Nicholas R, et al. Diabetic myonecrosis: likely an underrecognized entity. Orthopedics. 2014;37(10):e936-9.
3. Meher D, Mathew V, Misgar RM, et al. Diabetic Myonecrosis: An Indian Experience. Clinical Diabetes. 2013;31(2):53-8.

CASE 14: Cystic Fibrosis-related Diabetes

Satinath Mukhopadhyay, Partha Pratim Chakraborty

CASE HISTORY

A married young male in his early 30s referred for male factor infertility. He had been diagnosed with diabetes 3 years prior to his presentation and his family history was negative for diabetes in any first- or second-degree relatives. He had preserved libido, arousal and satisfactory penetration. He had no symptoms suggestive of pancreatic exocrine insufficiency or severe hyperglycemia. He had normal BMI (22.4 kg/m^2), normal testicular volume (25 mL) bilaterally without acanthosis nigricans.

Baseline investigations including fasting morning testosterone, luteinizing hormone (LH) and follicle-stimulating hormone (FSH) levels were within normal range. Abdominal ultrasound was normal. He had been put on sulfonylurea and metformin since diagnosis, with satisfactory glycemic control (FPG: 92 mg/dL, PPG: 132 mg/dL and HbA1c: 6.6%). Glucagon stimulated serum C-peptide level was 1.97 ng/mL (cut off: 1.8 ng/mL) and pancreatic autoantibodies (anti-GAD65 and anti-IA2 antibodies) were negative. Seminal fluid analysis was done thrice and each time it showed low ejaculate volume (<1 cc), low seminal fluid pH (<6.7), absent fructose and azoospermia. Because of persistent azoospermia and evidence suggestive of obstructive azoospermia (low ejaculate pH, volume and absent fructose), a transrectal ultrasound (TRUS) was performed which showed normal prostate with nonvisualization of seminal vesicles and vas deferentia bilaterally. With a working diagnosis of CF, sweat chloride test was advised. The sweat chloride level was >60 mEq/L on two occasions (77.7 mEq/L and 65.4 mEq/L, respectively).

DISCUSSION

Cystic fibrosis (CF) is caused by mutations in the CF transmembrane conductance regulator (CFTR) gene and transmitted in an autosomal recessive manner. The disease is characterized by abnormal chloride transport along the apical membrane of epithelial cells, culminating in progressive pulmonary and pancreatic dysfunction, elevated sweat chloride and male infertility. Instead of having involvement of all the said organs, individuals with atypical CF might have involvement of only one system, and symptoms/signs may remain subclinical adolescence or adulthood. For example the genitourinary abnormalities of CF are unveiled during evaluation of male factor infertility. Congenital absence of both the vas deferens (CABVD) simulates obstructive azoospermia on seminogram and CF should remain as an important differential diagnosis in such condition. Approximately half of adult CF patients develop cystic fibrosis-related diabetes (CFRD), that can manifest at any age. The mean age of diabetes onset is usually 18–21 years. Prevalence rates of CFRD increase with advancing age, and as many as 45–50% of adults >30 years of age may be affected. Pancreatic dysfunction, exocrine or endocrine can also be the primary presentation of CF. The progression of hyperglycemia is gradual and ketoacidosis is not common even in absence of insulin therapy. The pathophysiology of CFRD mimics that of fibrocalculous pancreatic diabetes (FCPD) and involves primarily insulin deficiency that is exacerbated by worsening insulin resistance secondary to recurrent infections.

Section 4: Diabetes

> **Take Home Messages**
> - Cystic fibrosis may have classic presentation with involvement of all the susceptible organs or the manifestation may subtle or atypical wherein respiratory, gastrointestinal, endocrine and genitourinary systems may be involved either alone or in varying combinations
> - Cystic fibrosis simulates obstructive azoospermia as evidenced by low ejaculate and absent fructose on semen analysis; acidic seminal fluid (pH <7.2) is an important clue to the underlying CFTR mutation
> - Many patients with CABVD may have CFTR mutations without overt signs/symptoms of CF and presence of CABVD is an indication for CFTR mutation study. They should be put on regular follow-up for potential late complications of CF like CFRD.

SUGGESTED READING

1. Moran A, Becker D, Casella SJ, et al. Epidemiology, pathophysiology, and prognostic implications of cystic fibrosis related diabetes: a technical review. Diabetes Care. 2010;33:2677-83.
2. Moran A, Brunzell C, Cohen R, et al. Clinical care guidelines for cystic fibrosis–related diabetes: a position statement of the American Diabetes Association and a clinical practice guideline of the Cystic Fibrosis Foundation, endorsed by the Pediatric Endocrine Society. Diabetes Care. 2010;33:2697-708.
3. Patrizio P, Asch RH. The relation between congenital absence of the vas deferens (CBAVD), cystic fibrosis (CF) mutations, and epididymal sperm. Assist Reprod Rev. 1994;4:95-100.

CASE 15: A Patient with Late Onset Diabetes in Adult

Satinath Mukhopadhyay, Partha Pratim Chakraborty

CASE HISTORY

A 32-year-old lady presented with uncontrolled hyperglycemia despite being on maximum daily dosages of glimepiride (8 mg), metformin (2 g) and pioglitazone (30 mg), 2 years after the onset of diabetes. She had presented to her primary care physician for polyuria, polyphagia, polydipsia, significant weight loss and fatigability started 14 months back. She was diagnosed to have diabetes and was put on oral antidiabetic agents. She had noticed significant improvement of her osmotic symptoms and her blood glucose values were within target range for the following 8 months. Then she had experienced progressive deterioration of glycemic control despite uptitrating her oral antidiabetic medications. Her family history is negative for diabetes. Her pregnancies were not complicated by GDM.

Findings on examination: Height: 160 cm, weight: 58 kg, BMI: 22.65 kg/m^2, waist = 72 cm, hip = 78.5 cm, waist/hip ratio = 0.91, BP: 110/80 mm Hg (supine), 104/78 mm Hg (standing) (right arm), ankle to brachial systolic blood pressure index (ABI): 1.05 (normal 0.9–1.3), pulse: 89 beats/min, regular, no radio-radial or radio-femoral delay. No acanthosis or lipoatrophy. Goiter: Grade 1b, fundus examination: No signs of DR. Monofilament 6/6 bilaterally, vibration perception threshold (VPT): Normal. Rest of the systemic examination was normal.

> **Investigations:** Hb%: 14.2 g%, TLC: 6,600/mm^3 (N72, L20), platelet: 2.5 lacs/mm^3, urea: 19, creatinine: 0.6, Na: 137, K: 3.9, SGOT: 36, SGPT: 67, albumin: 3.9, total cholesterol: 188 mg/dL, TGs: 105 mg/dL, HDL: 60 mg/dL, LDL: 107 mg/dL. LFT: Normal.
>
> Urine RE/ME: No pus cell, protein: Nil, ketone bodies: Nil.
>
> Fasting plasma glucose: 228 mg/dL, post breakfast plasma glucose: 326 mg/dL, HbA1c: 9.3%.
> - FT4: 0.96 ng/dL, TSH: 9.6 mIU/mL, TPO Ab: 96.5 IU/mL (<35)
> - ECG: Normal, USG abdomen: Liver, pancreas and kidneys are normal
> - Serum C-peptide: Fasting—0.76 ng/mL, stimulated (postglucagon)—1.64 ng/mL
> - GAD-65 antibody: 75.3 IU/mL (<10), IA-2 antibody: 63.5 IU/mL (<30)
> - tTg antibody (IgA): Negative, serum total IgA normal.

DISCUSSION

There are different classification systems of diabetes. The most widely accepted one, proposed by WHO and adopted by ADA, classifies diabetes into four subgroups: Type 1, Type 2, GDM and other specific types. Type 1 diabetes mellitus (T1DM) is of two types: 1a (with positive pancreatic autoimmune markers) and 1b (without pancreatic autoantibodies). From therapeutic point of view, however, the most relevant classification system is the Aβ system. Depending on presence/absence of pancreatic autoantibodies (A) and β-cell secretory reserve (β), diabetes can be subdivided into four groups: A+ β-, A+ β+, A- β+, A- β-. Autoimmune diabetes is a spectrum disorder with classical T1DM at one end and late onset autoimmune diabetes in adult (LADA) at the other. Unlike T1DM, LADA is seen in individuals in their 3rd or 4th decade. They initially respond to oral agents (≈6 months after diagnosis) and usually do not develop ketosis. The β-cell secretory reserve is poor (stimulated C-peptide <1.8 ng/mL) but they may not have absolute insulin deficiency (stimulated C-peptide <0.6 ng/mL). The pancreatic autoantibodies are positive and management of LADA is not different from the classical T1DM. LADA thus falls into A+ β- or A+ β+ subgroups of the Aβ classification system. Like Type 1a diabetes mellitus, patients of LADA may also have autoimmune polyendocrinopathy and should be screened for autoimmune thyroid disease and at times for celiac disease and Addison's disease. Patients of LADA do not have a family history of diabetes, are not obese and do not have clinical/biochemical features of insulin resistance. Absence of family history of diabetes and phenotypic and biochemical features of metabolic syndrome, i.e. truncal obesity, high BMI, acanthosis, skin tags, hypertension and diabetic dyslipidemia, characterized by high serum triacylglycerol and low serum HDL cholesterol, point toward a diagnosis of LADA, confirmed by presence of islet autoimmunity and usually, but not always, evidence of poor β-cell reserve at presentation.

> ### Take Home Messages
> - *Late onset diabetes in adult is a form of autoimmune diabetes usually seen in individuals in their 3rd or 4th decades*
> - *Patients are usually lean, have no family history of diabetes and do not have features of insulin resistance or diabetic dyslipidemia*
> - *They respond to oral agents for the initial few months and after that they become insulin dependent.*

SUGGESTED READING

1. Mollo A, Hernandez M, Marsal JR, et al. Latent autoimmune diabetes in adults is perched between type 1 and type 2: evidence from adults in one region of Spain. Diabetes Metab Res Rev. 2013;29(6):446-51.
2. Park Y, Hong S, Park L, et al. LADA prevalence estimation and insulin dependency during follow-up. Diabetes Metab Res Rev. 2011.;27(8):975-9.
3. Stenström G, Gottsäter A, Bakhtadze E, Berger B, Sundkvist G. Latent autoimmune diabetes in adults: definition, prevalence, beta-cell function, and treatment. Diabetes. 2005;54 (Suppl 2):S68-72.

CASE 16: Double Diabetes—But Differently Double

Soumyabrata Roy Chaudhuri

CASE HISTORY

A 30-year-old male was diagnosed as type 2 diabetes mellitus (T2DM) in December, 2014 was started on metformin initially and was then shifted on to glimepiride 4 mg and metformin 2 g/day and was under control. He became complacent and became irregular in follow-up.

In October 2017, he was admitted to the hospital with fever of 3 days duration with vertigo nausea, headache and bodyache. He stopped the antidiabetic drugs by himself from the 2nd day of fever. He was diagnosed to have dengue fever with low platelet counts and was treated with intravenous (IV) fluids, paracetamol and insulin was administered. He was eventually discharged on a basal bolus regimen. He was unable to walk postdischarge with leg pain and proximal muscle weakness was greater than that distal muscle. He took domiciliary physiotherapy sessions for a month and was gradually able to walk.

Over the next couple of months he was gradually weaned off the insulin and put back onto sulfonylurea, metformin and DPP4 inhibitor. He was admitted to the hospital again in May 2018 with pain abdomen, loss of weight and vomiting. The laboratory findings on admission are tabulated in Table 1.

He was referred for endocrine evaluation when he was asked for the C-peptide IAA and GAD antibodies (Table 2).

He was referred for endocrine evaluation when C-peptide IAA and GAD antibodies were ordered (Table 3).

He was referred for endocrine evaluation when he was asked for the C-peptide IAA and GAD antibodies. He was discharged on basal bolus insulin and followed up in OPD with the SMBG chart. His SMBG chart in his last visit in October 2018 is attached below in Table 4.

Treatment:
- LISPRO 10 U/10 U/10 U—before breakfast, lunch and dinner
- Glargine—32 U at 9 pm.

TABLE 1: Laboratory test reports 2017 (5 days after fever).

Parameters	Values
Serum, nonstructural protein 1	39.5 (Elisa)
Serum, IgM dengue	24.1 (Elisa)
Hemoglobin	14.1 g/dL
Platelets	28,500/mm^3
Packed cell volume	41.3%
Urine examination	
Albumin	+
Sugar	++
Acetone	++
Others	
Malaria antigen	Not found
HbsAg/HCV/HIV (1 and 2)	Nonreactive
Random sugar	269 mg/dL
Urea	29 mg/dL
Serum creatinine	1.2 mg/dL
Serum sodium	129 mEq/L
Serum potassium	4.2 mEq/L
SGOT/SGPT	205/213 U/L
Alkaline phosphatase	205 U/L

(HbsAg: hepatitis B surface antigen; HIV: human immunodeficiency virus; HCV: hepatitis C virus; SGOT: serum glutamic-oxaloacetic transaminase; SGPT: serum glutamic-pyruvic transaminase)

TABLE 2: Laboratory reports May 2018.

Parameters	Values
Glycosylated hemoglobin	12.3%
SGOT/SGPT	24/15 U/L
Alkaline phosphatase	138 U/L
Hemoglobin	14.8 g/dL
Total leukocyte count	14,550/mm^3
Platelets	1.8 lakhs/mm^3
Erythrocyte sedimentation rate	19 mm/h
Urine	Ketone bodies present

(SGOT: serum glutamic-oxaloacetic transaminase; SGPT: serum glutamic-pyruvic transaminase)

TABLE 3: Laboratory reports – 2018.

Parameters	Values
Glutamic acid decarboxylase antibody	+ (175.1)
C-peptide	0.2

TABLE 4: Capillary blood glucose reading.

Timing of test	Values
Before breakfast	162 mg/dL
Before lunch	217 mg/dL
Before dinner	255 mg/dL

DISCUSSION

Double diabetes is classically a combination of type 1 diabetes mellitus (T1DM) with features of insulin resistance and T2DM. The term "double diabetes" was first coined in 1991 based on the observation that patients with T1DM who had a family history of T2DM were more likely to be overweight and almost never achieved adequate glycemic control even with higher insulin doses. Stronger the family history the higher was the dose requirement which perhaps indicated the presence of increased resistance to insulin mediated glucose disposal in this subgroup of patients with T1DM.

Dengue fever is a mosquito-borne tropical disease and the most common arboviral illness in humans. Estimates suggest that approximately 50–528 million people are affected by the disease annually. A publication form Lahore reported that as many as 33% of the nondiabetic dengue patients having IgM positivity and platelet count of less than a lakh developed diabetes in this cohort. However, the hypothesis generated for this suggested activation of T lymphocytes an release of proinflammatory cytokines to be the main driver for this overlap as this activation leads to capillary leak in severe dengue and also fits with the inflammation hypothesis of etiopathogenesis of T2DM—in which the anatomical and physiological integrity of the endothelium is changed due to activation of the T lymphocytes.

However another publication from south India stated that as immune complex deposition in glomeruli could cause acute kidney injury in dengue, dengue-induced deposition of antigen and antibody complex in the Islets of Langerhans has also been documented and as such may be responsible for the pancreatitis and new onset diabetes documented in dengue patients. Coxsackievirus infection leading to T1DM is well known however this case possibly is a pointer that such possibility may also be true in case of dengue-infected subjects. In patients with new onset diabetes after dengue who remain uncontrolled or are difficult to control with OADS (oral antidiabetic agents), looking for C-peptide levels and autoantibodies for T1DM may be justified.

Take Home Message

- Sudden inability to control glycaemia with adequate oral anti diabetic agents following an episode of dengue fever should raise suspicion of autoimmune beta cell destruction.

SUGGESTED READING

1. Sudulagunta SR, Sodalagunta MB, Kumbhat M, et al. New Onset Diabetes Mellitus in Dengue Shock Syndrome. J Assoc Phys India. 2018;66:104.
2. Aamir M, Mukhtar F, Fatima A, et al. Newly Diagnosed Diabetes Mellitus in Patients with Dengue Fever Admitted in Teaching Hospital of Lahore. Diabetologia. 2013;56(7):1462-70.
3. Cleland SJ, Fisher BM, Colhoun HM, et al. Insulin resistance in type 1 diabetes: what is 'double diabetes' and what are the risks? Diabetologia. 2013;56(7):1462-70.

CASE 17: Diabetes Mellitus as Presenting Manifestation of Acromegaly due to Growth Hormone-secreting Pituitary Macroadenoma

Subhankar Chowdhury, Partha Pratim Chakraborty

CASE HISTORY

Patient A

A 42-year-old lady had been diagnosed with diabetes 3 years back and presented with uncontrolled hyperglycemia. A number of oral antidiabetic agents were prescribed in maximal dosage during the initial 2 years without effect and she was then switched to twice daily premixed insulin. Despite taking 64 IU of insulin (0.98 U/kg/day) and 2 g of metformin daily but her glycemic status was grossly deranged (FPG: 286 mg/dL; PPPG: 346 mg/dL; and HbA1c: 11.9%). Her family history was negative for diabetes and she had her last menstrual period 2 years back. She was otherwise asymptomatic.

Clinical evaluation revealed the following: Weight: 65 kg, height: 149.2 cm, body mass index (BMI): 29.1 kg/m², waist circumference: 94.5 cm, BP: 130/80 mm Hg, PR: 84 beats/min, neck vein: engorged and pulsatile, grade 2 acanthosis. A vigilant

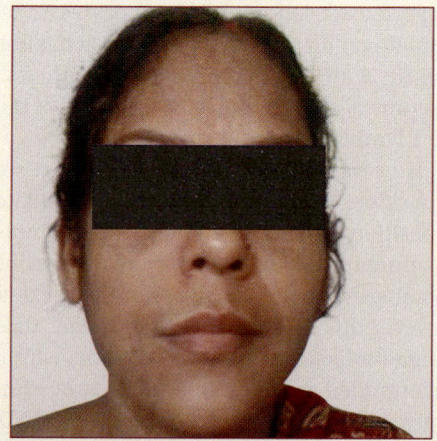

FIG. 1: Facial appearance of patient A.

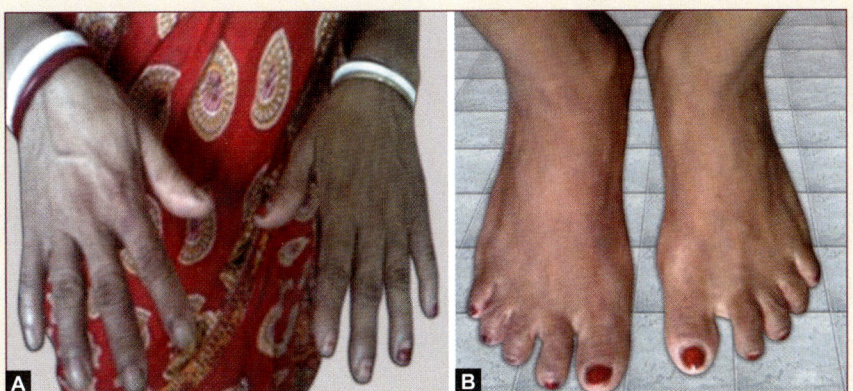

FIGS. 2A AND B: Hands of patient A.

examination also documented a subtle fleshy nose, thick lower lips, oily face, spade like hands, macroglossia (Figs. 1 and 2A and B). Rest of the systemic examination including confrontation perimetry was normal. Relevant investigations are summarized in Table 1.

Patient B

A 54-year-old gentleman consulted us with new onset diabetes (FPG: 169 mg/dL and PPPG: 321 mg/dL). He had no family history of diabetes. Apart from bilateral knee pain he was completely asymtomatic. Clinical examination revelaed normal BMI (22.9 kg/m^2), hypertension (BP: 154/104 mm Hg), broad and fleshy nose and spade-shaped hands (Figs. 3 and 4). Relevant investigations are summarized in Table 1.

TABLE 1: Summary of investigations.

Parameters	Patient A	Patient B
IGF-1	548 (normal: 98–261 ng/mL)	478 (normal: 84–233 ng/mL)
FT4 (normal: 0.8–1.8)	0.92 ng/dL	0.78 ng/dL
TSH (normal: 0.5–5)	0.81 mIU/L	5.7 mIU/L
Cortisol 8 AM (normal: 5–25)	18.61 µg/dL	4.8 µg/dL
FSH	0.66 mIU/mL	5.6 mIU/mL
Testosterone	–	157 ng/dL (normal: 300–900)
MRI pituitary (Figs. 5 and 6)	Pituitary macroadenoma with homogenous contrast enhancement	Enlarged sella, pituitary macroadenoma with minimal homogenous contrast enhancement

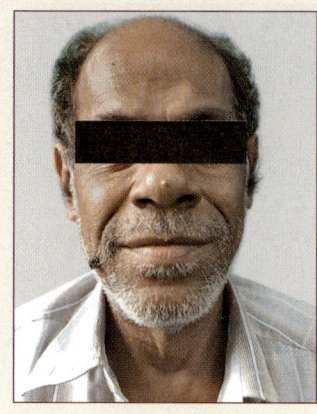

FIG. 3: Facial appearance of patient B.

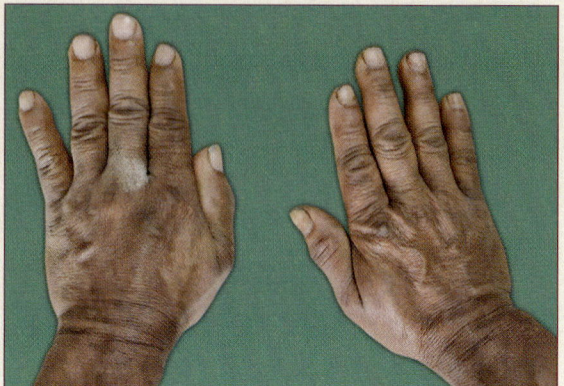

FIG. 4: Broad and spade-shaped hands of patient B.

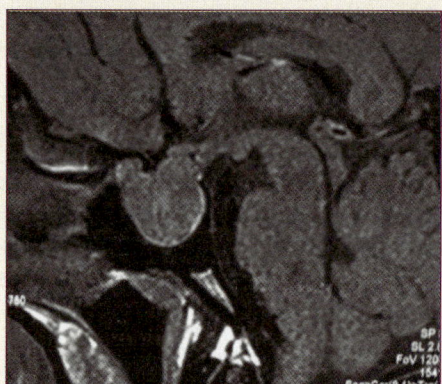

FIG. 5: MRI of patient A.

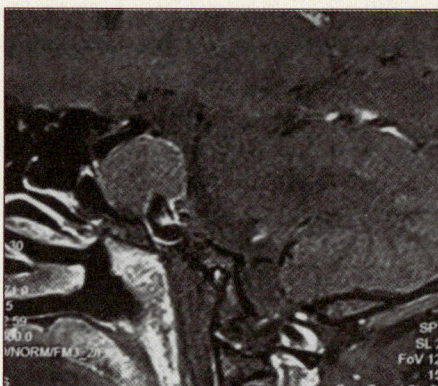

FIG. 6: MRI of patient B.

DISCUSSION

Acromegaly is caused by growth hormone secreting pituitary macroadenoma in majority of cases. Acromegaly is characterized by soft tissue and bony overgrowth like prognathism, broad and fleshy nose, macroglossia, thick lips, spade-shaped hands, increased heel pad thickness. However, these features are often overlooked and the mean delay in diagnosis is about 10 years after the estimated onset of symptoms. In a review of 164 patients with acromegaly, only 58 patients (35%) presented because of a change in features and 56 patients (34%) sought attention because of disturbances associated with acromegaly, including visual field defects, carpal tunnel syndrome and headaches. The remaining 50 patients had no complaints related directly to the acromegaly and were diagnosed when seeking medical consultation for an unrelated complaint. For an example, amenorrhea may be the most common presenting complaint in women. Insulin resistance is a frequent consequence of acromegaly. The prevalence of impaired glucose tolerance is up to 46% and type 2 diabetes mellitus is detected in up to 56% of patients with acromegaly. Hypertension is seen in up to 40% of patients. The presenting symptoms of acromegaly are of insidious onset and lack specificity. These include lethargy, headache and increased sweating; thus the diagnosis of acromegaly begins with a clinical suspicion and elevated IGF1 from the age and sex specific reference range. IGF1 can be measured at any time of the day irespective of food intake. The diagnosis is then confirmed by the nadir growth hormone (GH) suppression after administration of glucose, which is considered the "gold standard" test for acromegaly. The inability to suppress serum GH to less than 1 ng/mL after 75 g of glucose administration confirms the diagnosis. The next step in the diagnostic algorithm is MRI of pituitary. Anterior pituitary function should be evaluated in all patients with acromegaly by measuring prolactin, 8:00 AM. cortisol, FT4 and TSH. Hypogonadotropic hypogonadism is diagnosed by low fasting morning testosterone and low/normal FSH in males and low/normal FSH in amenorrheic females. The treatment of choice is surgery in almost all patients of acromegaly and such patients should be referred to an experienced surgeon after the diagnosis.

Take Home Messages

- *Type 2 diabetes mellitus is the most common type of adult onset diabetes mellitus. Secondary diabetes is encountered in a minority of adults with hyperglycemia and is often overlooked by the treating physician. Difficult to control hyperglycemia especially within a short period after diagnosis is an important clue to secondary diabetes*
- *Diagnosis of acromegaly is often missed particularly in individuals with subtle soft tissue and bony overgrowth. Broad and fleshy nose, thick lips, macroglossia, broad-shaped hands are the clinical clues to underlying hypersomatotropism*
- *Once the underlying condition is suspected, the diagnosis of acromegaly is confirmed with elevated IGF1, nonsuppressed GH after glucose load and pituitary imaging.*

SUGGESTED READING

1. Hanley NA. Endocrine disorders that cause diabetes. In: Holt RIG, Cockram CS, Flyvbjerg A, Goldstein BJ, eds. Textbook of Diabetes. 4th edn. Oxford: Wiley Blackwell, 2010:279-97.
2. Jadresic A, Banks LM, Child DF, et al. The acromegaly syndrome: relation between clinical features, growth hormone values and radiological characteristics of the pituitary tumours . Q J Med 1982;51(202): 189-204.
3. Katznelson L, Laws ER, Melmed S, et al. Acromegaly: an endocrine society clinical practice guideline. J Clin Endocrinol Metab. 2014;99:3933–51.

CASE 18
Diabetic Truncal Radiculoneuropathy: A Completely Reversible Form of Diabetic Neuropathy

Subhankar Chowdhury, Partha Pratim Chakraborty

CASE HISTORY

Two nonobese gentlemen in their mid-60s with long-standing type 2 diabetes mellitus noticed unilateral, dull-aching pain over the left side of their upper abdomen (involving the T7–T10 spinal segments) for preceding 2–4 months followed by appearance of a reducible swelling overlying the area (Figs. 1 and 2). Appearance of abdominal swelling prompted them to seek surgical consultation. Both of them had a documented weight loss of more than 5% over the previous 3 months and uncontrolled hyperglycemia (glycosylated hemoglobin levels were 11.2% and 10.1% respectively). They were referred to us with a diagnosis of left-sided lumbar hernia for preoperative glycemic control. Clinical examination revealed no underlying organomegaly and the swelling disappeared on lying in the right lateral decubitus position. They had diminished cutaneous sensations involving the left-sided T7–T10 dermatomes, distal symmetric peripheral small and large fiber neuropathy and moderate-to-severe nonproliferative diabetic retinopathy. Abdominal imaging was noncontributory.

In absence of any obvious cause of the abdominal swelling and presence of advanced microangiopathic complications in the background of long-standing uncontrolled diabetes, a diagnosis of diabetic truncal radiculoneuropathy with abdominal pseudohernia was considered which was confirmed subsequently by electrophysiological study.

Both patients were put on pregabalin and amitriptyline for pain relief and basal-bolus insulin regimen to optimize the blood glucose levels. Both of them improved symptomatically and self-monitoring of blood glucose revealed satisfactory values. Pregabalin and amitriptyline were gradually withdrawn. After 6 months of the initial presentation both patients noticed complete resolution of their abdominal swelling (Fig. 3). They had gained 10 kg each during this period and did not have pain or dysesthesia over the involved dermatomes. Cutaneous sensation (fine touch, crude touch and temperature) of the previously affected dermatome (T7–T10 segment on left side) returned back to normal.

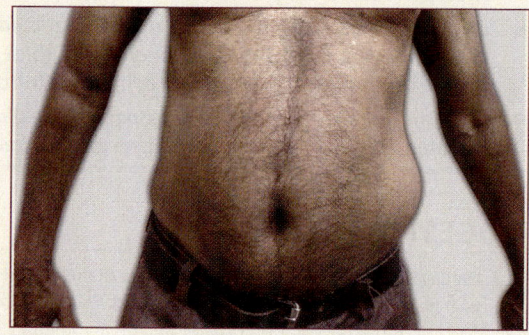

FIG. 1: Left-sided upper abdominal swelling misdiagnosed as lumbar hernia.

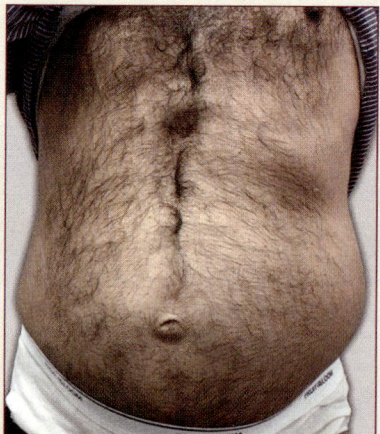

FIG. 2: Left-sided lumbar swelling and associated overlying muscle atrophy.

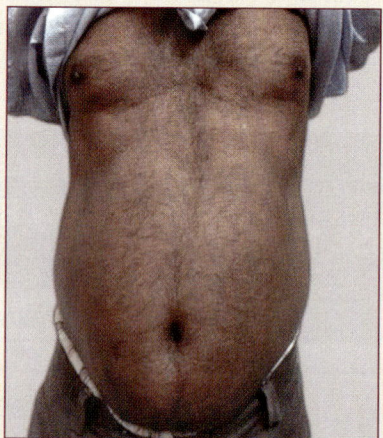

FIG. 3: Complete disappearance of the swelling at 6 months follow-up in one of them.

DISCUSSION

The true prevalence of truncal radiculoneuropathy in patients with diabetes is unknown and it has rarely been reported. Weight loss is a predominant feature and most of these patients have coexisting advanced microvascular complications of diabetes. Interestingly, duration of diabetes and glycemic status do not correlate with diabetic truncal radiculoneuropathy. The underlying pathophysiologic mechanism is still obscure, however, microinfarction and immune-mediated nerve damage have been proposed. Skin biopsies from the involved segment show loss of both epidermal and dermal nerve fibers. This particular form of diabetic neuropathy is self-limiting that usually resolves within months and has a favorable prognosis. Intraepidermal nerve fibers return after clinical recovery, suggesting that improvement occurs by neuronal regeneration. A minority of the patients may suffer from recurrent attacks of polyradiculopathy. Symptomatic relief from pain has been the mainstay of therapy. Efficacies of tricyclic antidepressants (TCAD) (e.g. amitriptyline), serotonin and noradrenaline reuptake inhibitors (SNRI) (e.g. duloxetine), calcium channel alpha-2-delta ligands (e.g. gabapentin, pregabalin) have been well established in neuropathic pain. Topical agents such as capsaicin and lidocaine are effective alternatives.

Take Home Messages

- *Diabetic truncal radiculoneuropathy, perhaps an underreported complication of diabetes is often overlooked and at times misdiagnosed by the physicians*
- *The patients should be counseled and reassured regarding the self-limiting nature of this entity*
- *Treatment of truncal radiculoneuropathy is completely symptomatic and judicious use of drugs for neuropathic pain along with satisfactory glycemic control usually gives good relief.*

SUGGESTED READING

1. Asbury AK. Focal and multifocal neuropathies of diabetes. In: Dyck PJ, Thomas PK, Asbury AK, et al, eds. Diabetic neuropathy. Philadelphia: Saunders. 1987:45-55.
2. Chiu HK, Trence DL. Diabetic neuropathy, the great masquerader: truncal neuropathy manifesting as abdominal pseudohernia. Endocr Pract. 2006;12(3):281-3.
3. Weeks RA, Thomas PK, Gale AN. Abdominal pseudohernia caused by diabetic truncal radiculoneuropathy. J Neurol Neurosurg Psychiatry. 1999;66(3):405.

CASE 19 | Acute Gastric Dilatation as Presenting Manifestation of Diabetic Ketoacidosis

Subhankar Chowdhury, Partha Pratim Chakraborty

CASE HISTORY

Patient A

An 11-year-old girl admitted to surgery emergency ward with recurrent vomiting for preceding 2 days associated with abdominal distension and ill-defined diffuse abdominal pain. She was profoundly dehydrated, cachectic and had tachycardia, hypotension and tachypnea with deep and labored respiration. Straight X-ray of the abdomen revealed a hugely dilated gastric shadow (Fig. 1). Baseline biochemistry documented hyperglycemia (445 mg/dL), hyponatremia (125 mEq/L) and high anion gap metabolic acidosis. Serum and urine ketones were strongly positive.

Patient B

A 13-year-old girl presented with repeated episodes of vomiting with epigastric fullness and generalized abdominal pain for 36 hours. She had malnutrition, severe dehydration and low grade fever. Her parents noticed that the girl had been suffering from polyuria and excessive thirst for the preceding 3 months. She had tachycardia (130 beats/min) with feeble peripheral pulses and nonrecordable blood pressure. Blood biochemistry documented elevated blood sugar (398 mg/dL), prerenal azotemia and high anion gap metabolic acidosis. Serum and urine ketones were elevated. Straight X-ray of abdomen revealed gastric dilatation (Fig. 2).

With a diagnosis of diabetic ketoacidosis (DKA), both the children were treated conservatively with nasogastric suction, intravenous fluids, insulin infusion, intravenous potassium and systemic antibiotics. Both of them responded favorably and were allowed oral feeding after 3 days of admission.

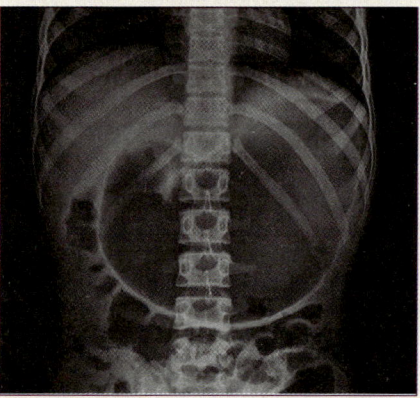 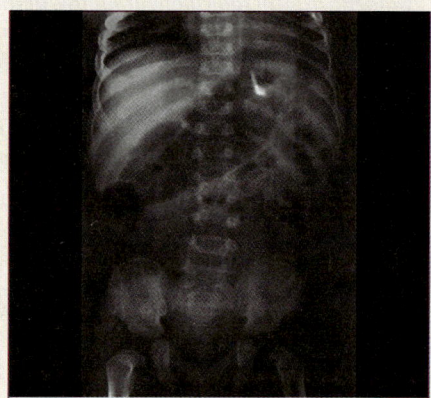

FIG. 1: Straight X-ray abdomen of patient A showing hugely distended stomach.

FIG. 2: Straight X-ray abdomen of patient B showing distended gastric shadow.

DISCUSSION

Diabetic ketoacidosis is an endocrine emergency in which profound insulin deficiency leads to hyperglycemia, excessive lipolysis with unrestrained fatty acid oxidation and resultant excess ketone production. This results in high anion gap metabolic acidosis, dehydration and deficits in body fluids and electrolytes. The proposed pathogenesis of the reversible gastrointestinal manifestations (nausea, vomiting, abdominal pain and distension), which frequently accompany DKA is multifactorial, involving metabolic, humoral, microvascular and neural processes. Insulin deficiency itself along with elevated circulating levels of glucagon, catecholamines and other hormones accompanying DKA impede gastrointestinal motility and result in gastric atony and generalized ileus. Hyperglycemia per se has also been implicated in interfering with gastrointestinal motility. Even bacterial toxins from concurrent respiratory tract or systemic infections may inhibit gastric motility and precipitate this event. The abdominal symptoms secondary to DKA alone usually resolve completely following improvement of the metabolic abnormalities.

Severe gastroparesis is potentially hazardous in these patients as it increases the risk of aspiration of gastric contents in individuals with altered sensorium. It is also responsible for poor and erratic glycemic control following enteral feeding due to a discrepancy between the onset of insulin action and release of nutrients into the small intestine. On rare occasions, acute gastric dilatation may be the sole presenting manifestation of DKA. Such physical sign that suggests an acute surgical abdomen may lead to unnecessary hazardous surgical interventions in patients with previously undiagnosed diabetes. Moreover, a delay in diagnosis and institution of appropriate therapy in DKA significantly increases the case fatality rate in children.

To conclude, primary nonabdominal causes of acute gastric dilatation should also be considered in children presenting with abdominal distension and recurrent vomiting who are malnourished, hypotensive and hyperventilating.

Take Home Messages

- *Gastrointestinal symptoms are quite common in patients with DKA, frequently dominate the clinical picture and act as potential "red herring" leading to delay in appropriate management*
- *Clinicians should be able to differentiate gastrointestinal symptoms secondary to DKA from those caused by a primary intra-abdominal process which has an entirely different therapeutic connotation*
- *Gastrointestinal manifestations of DKA resolve completely with resolution of the metabolic disturbances following appropriate treatment with fluids, insulin and electrolytes.*

SUGGESTED READING

1. Barrett EJ, Sherwin RS. Gastrointestinal manifestations of diabetic ketoacidosis. Yale J Biol Med. 1983;56(3):175-8.
2. Dragstadt LR, Montogomery ML, Ellis JC, Matthews WB. The pathogenesis of acute dilatation of the stomach. Surgery, Gynecology and Obstetrics. 1931;52:1075-86.
3. Valerio D. Acute diabetic abdomen in childhood. Lancet. 1976;1(7950):66-8.

CASE 20 | A Patient where Continuous Glucose Monitoring System Helped

Sudip Chatterjee

CASE HISTORY

Mr AM, a 64-year-old male had type 2 diabetes mellitus for the last 26 years. He was first seen in March 2010 and started on glimepiride, vildagliptin and metformin. The doses of the oral agents were gradually increased and ultimately he had to be started on insulin from October 2010. He was given lispro mix 25/75, 28 units before breakfast and 24 units before dinner together with pioglitazone. He was reasonably controlled with HbA1c of 7.8%. In August 2012, when the HbA1c was 8.5%, he was put on lispro before breakfast and lunch and his usual lispro mix before dinner. He had monomorphic VPS's for which no action was taken.

The patient returned after 4 years in August 2016 with features of foot neuropathy. He had stopped lispro and had gone back to twice daily premix and HbA1c was 8.4. The patient came back in August 2017 and was taking premix 25/75 three times a day on his own. He reported a FBG of 70–90 mg/dL on most days and a 2-hour post lunch value of 100–130 mg/dL. However his HbA1c was 8.1. This value was too high to match with the reported FBG and 2 hours PPBG. There was no evidence of thalassemia or variant hemoglobin. The patient was quite confident of his readings and denied any episodes of hypoglycemia. I felt that the best way to resolve this seeming mismatch was to do continuous glucose monitoring. Continuous glucose monitoring system (CGMS) was done in April 2018. This showed that the glucose values were high all night and just touched the baseline (Fig. 1) in the morning and 2 hours after lunch. In fact the only two times the glucose values were low normal, were the fasting value and the 2 hours post lunch value measured at 2 PM. At all other times the values were high. The insulin doses were adjusted taking this new finding into account.

The patient was last seen in November 2018. HbA1c was 7.7. He was distraught due to recent death of his wife. However he felt much better and seemed to have more energy. He felt that his HbA1c was slightly high due to the stress of his personal tragedy.

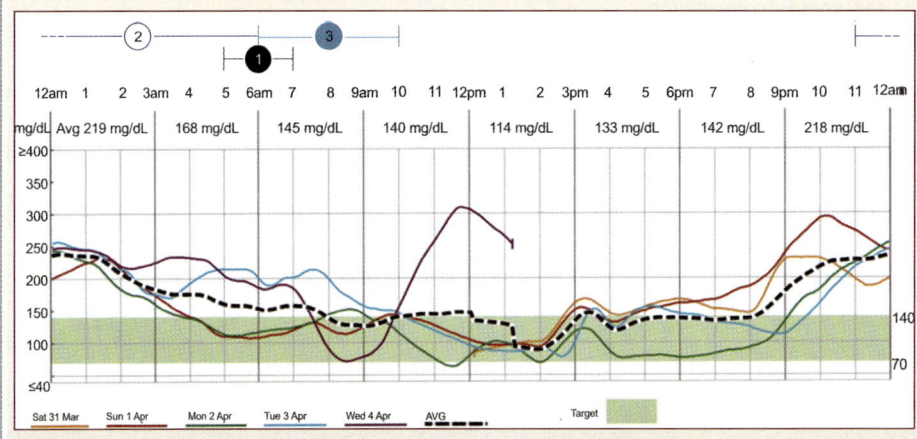

FIG. 1: CGMS values of this patient.

DISCUSSION

There are many occasions where the glycosylated hemoglobin is higher than would be expected from the patient's recent fasting or postprandial glucose values. The commonest reason for this is that most patients become more adherent to their meal and medication just before they are scheduled to see their doctor. Other causes can operate as well, which

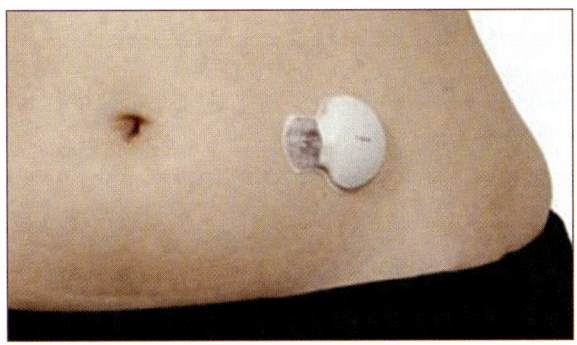

FIG. 2: The continuous glucose monitoring system sensor.

are outside the patient's control. For example undetected hemoglobinopathies can give a spuriously high HbA1c value. High performance liquid chromatography (HPLC) of the hemoglobin can diagnose β-thalassemia trait and many abnormal hemoglobins. It does not however pick up α-thalassemia carriers. There can be rare carbamylation defects of the hemoglobin that cause abnormally high HbA1c in spite of normoglycemia. In this patient CGMS clearly showed where the problem lay. Often the physician assumes that all cases of mismatch between glucose values and the HbA1c are due to poor adherence. There are many instances where this assumption does not hold true, as shown in this particular example. The CGMS device available to us (Fig. 2) is small and simple to use anc can record interstitial fluid glucose every 5 minutes for up to 7 days, but needs 12 hourly calibration using finger stick glucose.

Take Home Messages

- *It is quite common to have a mismatch between the HbA1c and the recorded blood glucose values, especially if the latter have been measured in a laboratory. Usually this is due to patient related factors like misreporting the values or adopting a more stringent diet and exercise routine just before the test. Variant hemoglobins can sometimes cause a problem*
- *In this case the decision to listen to the patient paid off. The patient was in the habit of taking an early lunch at 12 noon and he was taking lispro mix 25/75 before breakfast, lunch and dinner. This probably accounted for his unusual CGMS pattern*
- *Usage of aspart mix 30/70, three times a day has been documented in the literature as a useful way of controlling diabetes. The lunch time dose has to be kept low, however. It was reasonable to allow the patient to continue with his three times a day lispro mix routine with some adjustments. This is because aspart mix 30/70 and lispro mix 25/75 are very similar products*
- *CGMS systems measure interstitial fluid glucose which has a lag time of 4–26 minutes behind capillary glucose. The manufacturer states that the information is intended to supplement not replace readings from a home glucose monitor. Further, these systems give an indication when the patient should obtain a reading from a home glucose meter and give information regarding potential high and low glucose levels*
- *In spite of these caveats, CGMS provides useful information which translates into better patient care.*

SUGGESTED READING

1. Susana R Patton and Mark A Clements. Continuous Glucose Monitoring Versus Self-monitoring of Blood Glucose in Children with Type 1 Diabetes- Are there Pros and Cons for Both? US Endocrinol. 2012;8(1): 27-9.
2. Fonda SJ, Walker MS, Salkind SJ, Vigersky RA. Advantages and Disadvantages of Realtime Continuous Glucose Monitoring in People with Type 2 Diabetes. US Endocrinology. 2012;8(1):22-6.

CASE 21: A Patient with Interesting Problems
Sudip Chatterjee

CASE HISTORY

A 67-year-old woman with diabetes for 14 years was on aspart mix 30 twice daily. This was given by her son. The patient had rheumatoid arthritis which had gone into remission but had left her with deformities and poor power in the thumbs. She was unable to use syringes or the pen device she was prescribed. Control was poor as her son was a busy professional and unable to inject insulin at appropriate time. All the available insulin pen devices were evaluated. It was found that the Humalog disposable Kwikpen was the only device she could use independently. Changing to this device immediately resulted in a fall of her HbA1c from 9.4% to 8.3% over 4 months.

The patient then complained of severe night cough with loss of sleep and stress incontinence. On examination, the chest was clear and she was afebrile. The chest X-ray was normal. She was not on angiotensin-converting enzyme (ACE) inhibitors or angiotensin receptor blockers. She was advised to have an upper gastrointestinal (GI) endoscopy but refused. A barium meal examination of the stomach was done. In the upright position the study was normal. However when she was placed in the head down

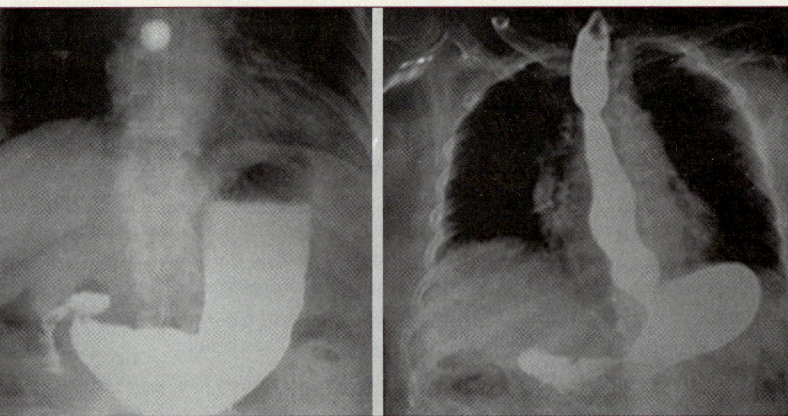

FIG. 1: The patient's barium meal of the stomach. The second radiograph taken in the Trendelenburg position shows severe gastroesophageal reflux.

or Trendelenburg position, there was severe reflux of barium all the way to the lower end of the pharynx.

Once the cause of cough was established, endoscopic fundoplication was discussed with the patient. However we could not locate a single center carrying out this procedure in Eastern India. The patient was unwilling to travel. Simple management measures were suggested like having an early dinner and leaving a long gap between the evening meal and bedtime. She was asked to raise the head end of her bed and take itopride 150 mg twice daily. She reported a slight improvement in her symptoms and was content to leave it at that. Complete resolution of this problem was not therefore possible.

DISCUSSION

This patient brings out several interesting facets of management of real life patients.
1. Insulin injection should be done either by the patient of a close family member, not by a compounder. It is worth exploring in details the barriers a patient may have in doing self injection. In this patient she did not have adequate power in her right thumb to push the plunger of the insulin pen she was using. Once a pen was identified where the pressure needed was less, she happily managed self injection
2. A chronic cough can have many causes. Achalasia cardia and gastro-esophageal reflux can cause overspill, mediastinitis and cough. A high index of suspicion is needed to make a diagnosis
3. Sharing decision making with the patient is now the norm. This patient was entirely satisfied with the autonomy a new insulin pen gave her. The fact that her cough had a cause gave her enormous satisfaction. She had no desire to go for treatment for the reflux
3. Endoscopic fundoplication is the current standard of care, as opposed to open or surgical fundoplication. There are very few centers in India that offer this service, because of the rarity of the condition.

Take Home Messages

- *There are two unrelated issues in this patient. Patients with rheumatoid disease affecting the thumb may find it difficult if not impossible to self-inject insulin. The pen devices of the different manufacturers require varying amounts of finger pressure to discharge the insulin. Of all the pens available in the market, there was only one pen that this patient could use independently. Changing over to that pen made a significant difference to her diabetes control*
- *Achalasia cardia and reflux esophagitis are recognized causes of prolonged coughing. Neither may show up on a plain chest X-ray. Upper GI endoscopy or barium studies can pick up the condition, provided there is initially an index of suspicion. The patient had all treatment options explained to her, but she ultimately decided to do nothing about it.*

SUGGESTED READING

1. Richardson T, Kerr D. Skin-related complications of insulin therapy: epidemiology and emerging management strategies. Am J Clin Dermatol. 2003;4(10):661-7.
2. Insulin Administration, American Diabetes Association Diabetes Care. 2004;27(suppl 1): s106-s107. https://doi.org/10.2337/diacare.27.2007.S106.
3. Irwin RS, French CL, Curley FJ, et al. Chronic cough due to gastroesophageal reflux: clinical, diagnostic, and pathogenetic aspects. Chest. 1993;104:1511-7.

SECTION 5

Diabetic Foot

CASE 1: A Case of Acute Charcot's Joint
Debmalya Sanyal

CASE HISTORY

A 59-year-old diabetic male patient presented with gradual swelling of the left foot for last 3 months. The swelling was not posture dependent. There was no history of fever, pain or any major trauma on the left foot. He was suffering from type 2 diabetes mellitus (T2DM) for the last 19 years and was on insulin therapy for the last 1 year. His HbA1c was 8.7%, he had tingling and numbness of both feet for last 5 years.

On examination his left ankle and foot was swollen with overlying dry and shiny skin. There were multiple areas of bony swelling over the tarsometatarsal and metatarsophalangeal joints with features of synovial effusion. Painless bony crepitus was also felt on palpation over the metatarsophalangeal joints with maximum crepitus over the left 5th metatarsophalangeal joint. Most of the tarsometatarsal and metatarsophalangeal joints were grossly disorganized, unstable but movement of the left ankle joint was preserved in most directions with very little pain while passive movement. Dorsalis pedis and posterior tibial artery pulses were normally palpable on the left side.

The X-ray of the left ankle joint revealed grossly disorganized and malaligned tarsal bone, bony swelling of the phalangeal ends of the metatarsal bones (especially the 2nd and 3rd metatarsophalangeal joints), fracture of the 5th metatarsal joint and dislocation of the 5th metatarsophalangeal joint with distinct joint margins. Based on the clinical features and investigations, the patient was diagnosed as a case of left Charcot's (neuropathic) joints predominantly involving the tarsal and metatarsal bones, tarsometatarsal and metatarsophalangeal joints. His total and differential counts were normal.

Diabetes mellitus is the most common cause of neuropathic joint disease. The term Charcot's joint is used interchangeably with neuropathic joints. Other rarer causes of Charcot's joint are syringomyelia, leprosy, Charcot-Marie-Tooth disease, amyloidosis, etc. In syringomyelia mostly the upper limb joints like glenohumeral, elbow or wrist are affected while in diabetes mellitus lower limb joints like tarsal or tarsometatarsal joints are affected.

Radiographic study in neuropathic joints reveals reduced joint spaces, subchondral sclerosis, joint effusion, osteophyte, grossly destroyed joints and hypertrophic changes. Fractures, extra-articular bone formations, bone resorption are noted in advanced cases. A close differential diagnosis is osteomyelitis but in osteomyelitis joint margins are indistinct and Indium-111 bone scan shows an increased uptake.

ACTIVE CHARCOT

The occurrence of neuropathic joint in diabetes is around 0.5%. Intense dynamic Charcot neuro-osteoarthropathy is characterized by clinical signs. There ought to be neuropathy and a warm and swollen foot. The skin temperature ought to be 2°C or more at the site of most extreme disfigurement of the influenced foot contrasted and a comparable site on the contralateral foot. The differential finding is disease (osteomyelitis, cellulitis and septic joint pain), irritation (gout, rheumatoid joint pain) and profound vein thrombosis. In this beginning time radiographic variations from the norm are absent.

OSTEOMYELITIS VERSUS CHARCOT

In contrast to osteomyelitis, Charcot neuro-osteoarthropathy is principally an articular sickness, which is most generally situated in the midfoot. In the beginning period radiography will not exhibit bone variations from the norm, yet MRI will indicate subchondral bone marrow edema. The subcutaneous delicate tissues are very little included. Signal forces on MRI will not segregate between dynamic Charcot joint or osteomyelitis.

Areas, e.g., bone or joint and ulcer or not, are the signs to the correct analysis. The intense phase of Charcot neuro-osteoarthropathy demonstrates quick and dynamic bone and joint devastation inside days or weeks. Fixed status by all out contact throwing can counteract further bone and joint decimation. X-ray pictures of a patient with intense Charcot neuro-osteoarthropathy (Fig. 1). The bone marrow edema ordinarily is not limited to a couple of bones yet is found in the whole midfoot. Bone marrow edema and its upgrade are regularly focused in the subchondral bone proposing articular illness. The subcutaneous tissues are moderately typical and there is no ulcer or different indications of disease.

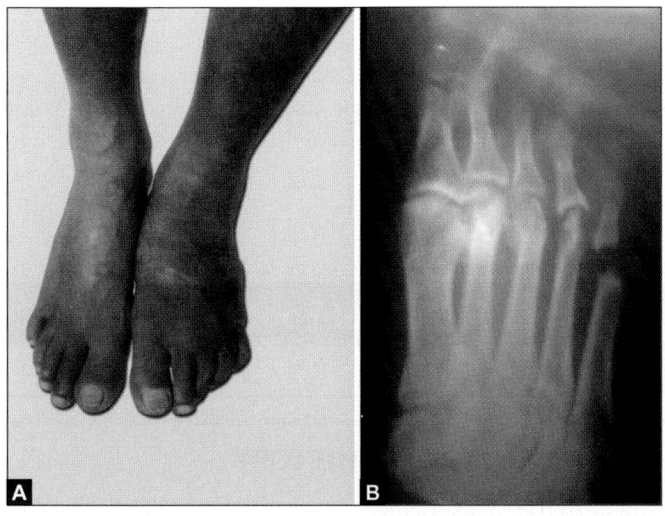

FIGS. 1A AND B: Image and X-ray of acute Charcot of left foot.

OSTEOMYELITIS

Osteomyelitis ought to be barred and fever is absent. Osteomyelitis in a diabetic with neuropathy is disease of the bone that typically results from adjacent spread of a skin ulcer. Therefore, the most widely recognized area for osteomyelitis is not in the midfoot, however at the weight purposes of the forefoot (metatarsal heads, IP joints) and in the hindfoot at the plantar part of the back calcaneus. Serum C-receptive protein level is typical or just a somewhat raised. To decide if osteomyelitis is available, is to put a marker on the ulcer or sinus tract and track it down deep and assess the MR-signal power of the marrow. Treatment of Charcot's joint is mostly unsatisfactory. Primary focus of treatment is stabilization of the joint, off loading and bisphosphonates. This patient was treated with off-loading and bisphosphonates.

DISCUSSION

Neuropathic osteoarthropathy is a moderately uncommon foot problem in diabetes but can have serious results. Though nearly 50% of patients with diabetes have polyneuropathy only 1% have Charcot. Trauma, osteitis and medical procedure inside the foot can be activating elements.

Fringe nerve damage and rehashed microinjuries lead to microfractures along with bone and articular structure degeneration. Because of proprioceptor harm, the foot ends up helpless to rehashed and undiscovered wounds. Proinflammatory cytokines, for example, IL-6, IL-1 and TNF-α, factor κB ligand (RANKL) add to the separation of develop osteoclasts aggravate bone erosion.

> **Take Home Message**
>
> - The characteristic feature of acute Charcot arthropathy is a warm and swollen foot in the background of diabetes polyneuropathy. The clinical picture impersonates conditions like osteomyelitis, cellulitis, e.g. a gout assault or profound vein thrombosis. But in Charcot there is no sinus tract and MRI may be helpful for early differentiation.

SUGGESTED READING

1. Shlomo Melmed, Kenneth Polonsky, P. Reed Larsen, Henry Kronenberg "Williams Textbook of Endocrinology, 13th edition, 2015, Elsevier.

CASE 2: A Case of Charcot Foot
Ghanshyam Goyal

CASE HISTORY

A 44-year-old male with poorly controlled type 2 diabetes mellitus (T2DM) attended the diabetic foot clinic with painless, hot, swollen and red left foot (Fig. 1).

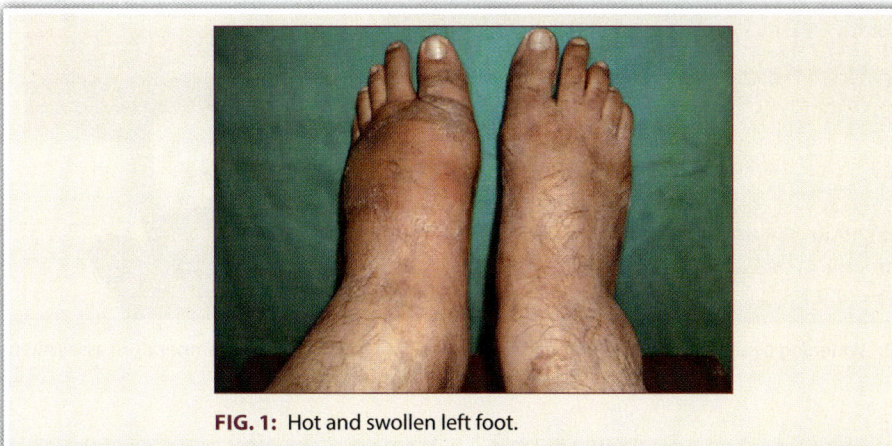

FIG. 1: Hot and swollen left foot.

DISCUSSION

Case History and Management

Charcot's osteoarthropathy is one of the major complications of diabetes. Factors that accelerate this process are peripheral neuropathy, increase in local blood flow, unrecognized injury and repetitive stress. This condition is characterized by pathological fractures, joint dislocation and destruction of architecture of the foot. Increased foot temperature is the first sign of inflammation in an insensate foot. Skin temperature assessment with an infrared thermometer and showing a temperature difference of more than 2°C as compared to the contralateral foot should raise a suspicion of charcot foot. Patients suspected to charcot joint should be immediately immobilized unless other causes have been established.

Charcot arthropathy should be suspected if there is redness, warmth, swelling or deformity (in particular, when the skin is intact), especially in the presence of peripheral neuropathy or renal failure. Think about acute Charcot arthropathy even when deformity is not present or pain is not reported.

Differential diagnosis of cellulitis, osteomyelitis, gout and deep vein thrombosis should be excluded.

We should also be aware that if a person with diabetes fractures his foot or ankle, it may progress to Charcot arthropathy.

Monofilament and VPT were grossly impaired. On examination both dorsalis pedis and posterior tibial arteries were palpable in both feet.

Ankle/Brachial index: Right 0.9 and left 1.0.

X-ray of foot shows widening of angle between 1st and 2nd metatarsal (MT) head (Fig. 2). Temperature of both feet measured with infrared thermometer and left foot is 3°C hotter than the right foot (Fig. 3).

The handheld infrared thermometer is a useful tool in predicting the risk of future ulceration in a neuropathic foot and studies have shown that self-monitoring of skin temperature may reduce the risk of ulceration.

A diagnosis of Charcot foot was made and the patient was advised immediate immobilization with total contact cast (TCC). The patient and the family members refused as they believed that since the patient had no fracture and hence the patient did not require TCC. We tried to counsel them that TCC was highly recommended for him to

Case Studies in Diabetology and Endocrinology

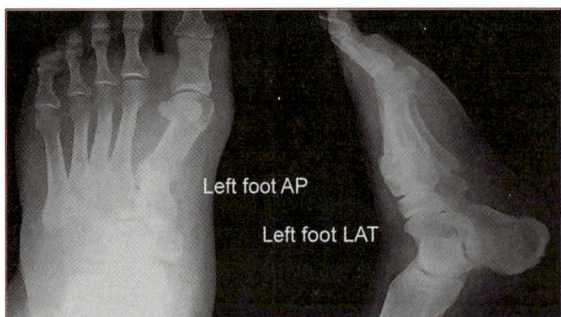

FIG. 2: Widening of angle between 1st and 2nd MT head.

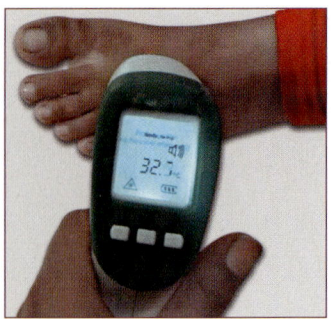

FIG. 3: Foot temperature assessment.

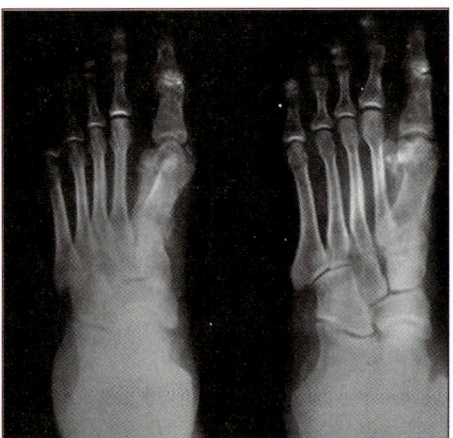

FIG. 4: X-ray showing fracture at 1st MT head.

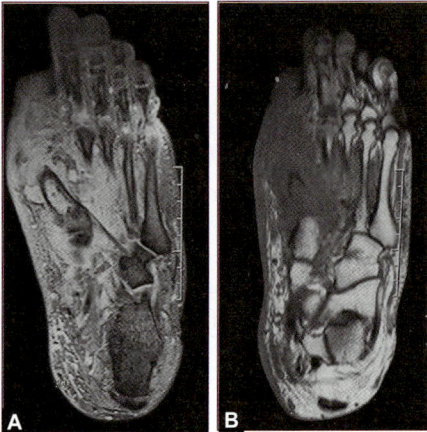

FIGS. 5A AND B: MRI showing Charcot changes.

save the limb from further damage but the patient was not convinced. Finally the patient was asked to get an MRI of the foot done.

The NICE guidelines recommend an MRI if the X-ray is normal but Charcot arthropathy is still suspected.

After 17 days he returned to foot clinic with increased swelling and redness. He was advised repeat X-ray of foot which shows fracture of 1st MT and disruption of tarsal bones (Fig. 4).

MRI of the foot was done which revealed charcot changes (Figs. 5A and B).

Patient was given total contact cast (Fig. 6) which was changed every 3 weeks. After 12 weeks the TCC was removed and the patient was put on posterior slab (is an easy-to-use, preassembled synthetic splinting system). Made from polyurethane coated fiberglass covered by polypropylene padding, which provides stabilization in 2–4 minutes and enables weight bearing in just 20 minutes.

Since posterior slab is removable the patient and family were made to understand the need of strict adherence to the offloading modality. Foot temperature was measured on every visit. After 16 weeks, temperature difference between both feet was less than 2°C and patient was put on "ankle foot orthosis" (Fig. 7) and advised regular follow-up (Figs. 8 and 9).

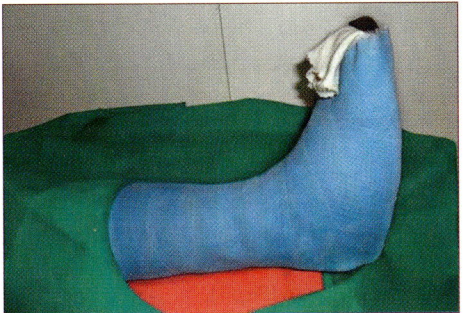

FIG. 6: Total contact cast.

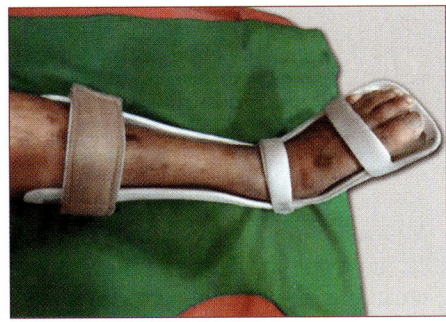

FIG. 7: Ankle foot orthosis.

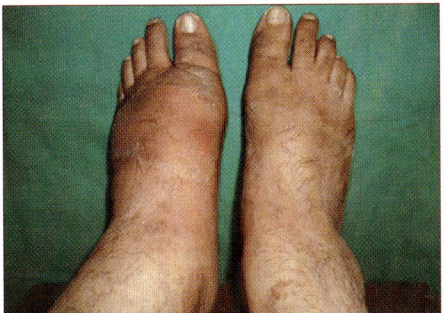

FIG. 8: At presentation.

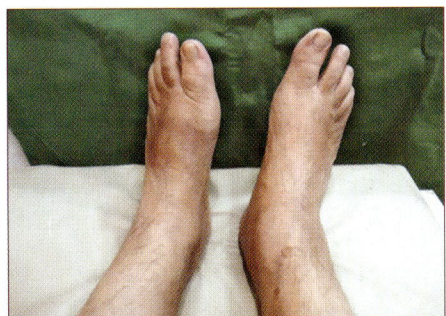

FIG. 9: After 4 months.

Take Home Messages

- *Strong suspicion in context of clinical picture and early immobilization with TCC is the key to successful management of Charcot foot. Early intervention prevents deformities*
- *Need for compliance with offloading modality should be stressed upon on every visit. These patients should be on lifelong surveillance.*

SUGGESTED READING

1. Lavery LA, Higgins KR, Lanctot DR, et al. Preventing diabetic foot ulcer recurrence in high-risk patients: Use of temperature monitoring as a self-assessment tool. Diabetes Care. 2007;30(1):14-20.
2. NICE (National Institute for Health and Care Excellence). (2019). Foot care for people with diabetes. [online] Available from http://pathways.nice.org.uk/pathways/foot-care-for-people-with-diabetes. [Last accessed May, 2019].
3. Rogers LC, Frykberg RG, Amstrong DG, et al. The Charcot foot in diabetes. Diabetes Care. 2011;34(9): 2123-9.

CASE 3: Ischemic Diabetic Foot

Ghanshyam Goyal

CASE HISTORY

A 70-year-old male, type 2 diabetes mellitus (T2DM) 20 years, body mass index (BMI) of 19 and history of coronary artery bypass grafting (CABG), presented with blackening of great, 2nd and 5th toe of right foot for 6 weeks with severe pain (Fig. 1).

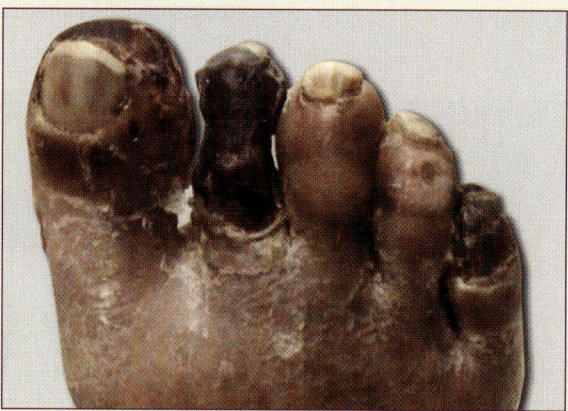

FIG. 1: Blackening of toes.

DISCUSSION

Case History and Management

Whenever a diabetic patient reports to a diabetic foot clinic, a comprehensive foot screening should be performed which includes sensation, vascularity, deformity, areas of pressure, footwear, and skin and signs of infection. Assessment of risk factors is also mandatory. Blood sugar levels, physical activity, smoking and or other forms of tobacco use, trauma and footwear are all modifiable risk factors whereas neuropathy, bony deformity, peripheral artery disease (PAD), previous history of ulceration and or amputation and age are nonmodifiable risk factors. Examination revealed dry gangrene of great, 2nd and 5th toe.

Palpation of pedal pulses is mandatory in any patient presenting with DFU. The ankle/brachial index (ABI) is the first noninvasive test that should be performed to check vascular status. One should remember that ABI may be falsely elevated in diabetic patients with calcified foot arteries. In these patients toe pressure and transcutaneous oxygen tension ($TcPO_2$) should be measured. Both dorsalis pedis and posterior tibial pulses were absent (Fig. 2).

Ankle/brachial index: Right 0.63 and left 0.62.

Vascular status: All patients with diabetes irrespective of whether a foot ulcer is present or not should be evaluated for PAD. PAD is a significant risk factor for development of diabetic foot ulcer (DFU). PAD is four times more common in people with diabetes

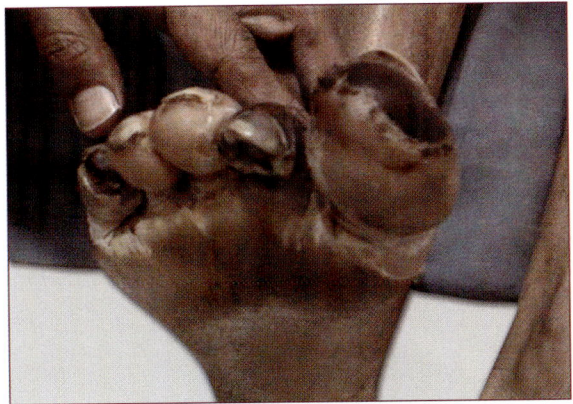

FIG. 2: Palpation of pedal pulses.

as compared to nondiabetics. It is estimated that 50% of patients with DFU will have significant PAD.

Doppler study of both lower limbs arteries revealed atherosclerotic grade II vessels. Angiography of peripheral limb was performed which revealed—Right: Complete block—no distal runoff and left: Complete block—adequate distal runoff.

- Angioplasty with stenting to right superficial femoral artery done (Fig. 3)
- Postangioplasty ABI improved and was: Right 0.93 and left 0.98.

Amputation of 2nd and 5th toe and partial amputation of great toe done (Fig. 4). Regular dressings and medical management continued.

- Ultrasonic debridement done (Fig. 5) and 2nd and 5th toe treated with regular dressing
- Disarticulation of great toe was performed
- Patient had severe rest pain and ulcers were still nonhealing.

In view of rest pain and nonhealing of ulcer repeat ABI was done which showed—Right 0.69 and left 0.80.

- Peripheral angiography performed which revealed: In-stent stenosis
- Balloon dilatation and drug balloon (peclitexel) done (Fig. 6)
- Regular dressings and medical management continued
- Repeat ABI was done which revealed improvement with: Right 1.04 and left 0.82
- Posterior slab was given and regular dressings continued (Figs. 7 and 8).

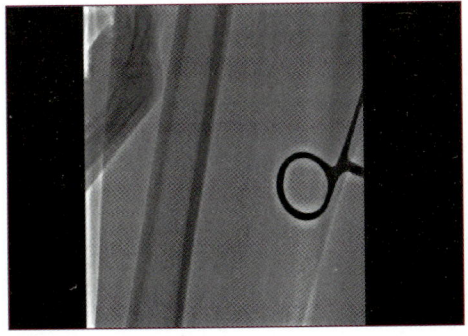

FIG. 3: Angioplasty with stenting.

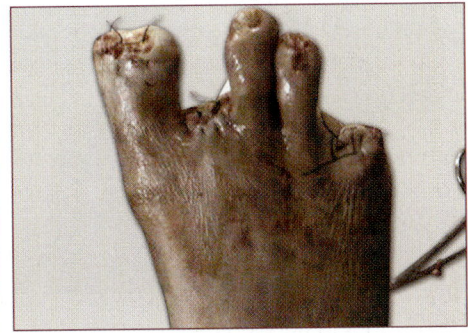

FIG. 4: Post amputation.

Gradually the ulcers healed. Patient was kept on posterior slab for a month after healing of ulcers (Figs. 9 and 10).

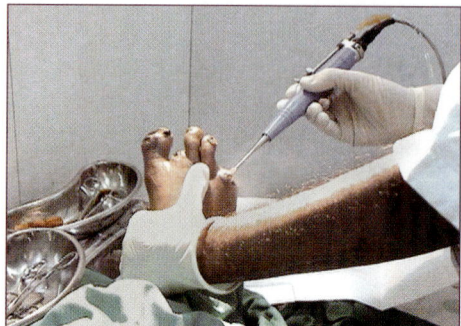

FIG. 5: Ultrasonic debridement of wound.

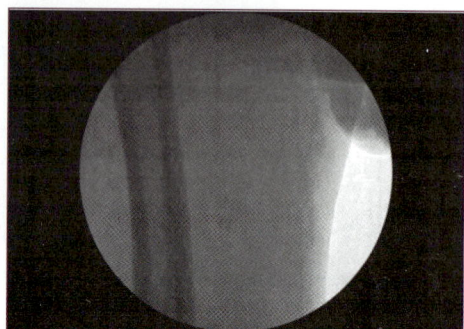

FIG. 6: Balloon dilatation.

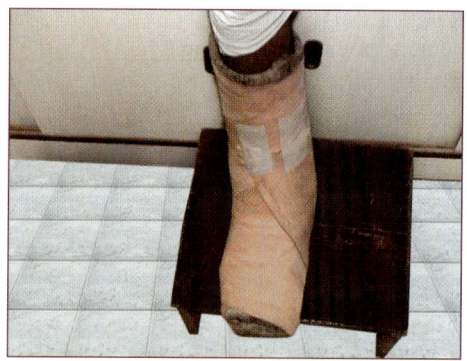

FIG. 7: Posterior slab.

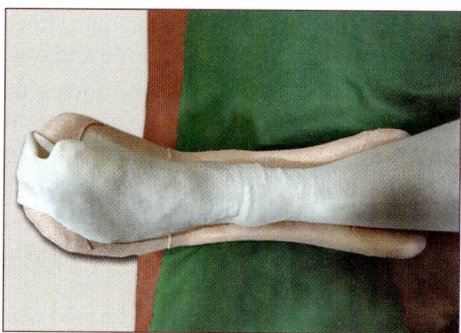

FIG. 8: Posterior slab.

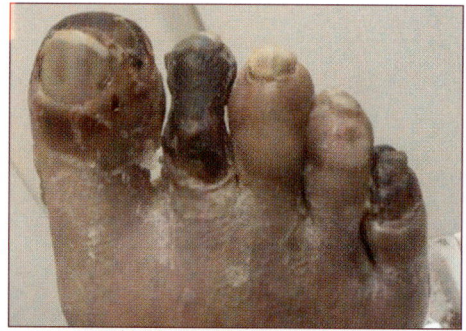

FIG. 9: At presentation.

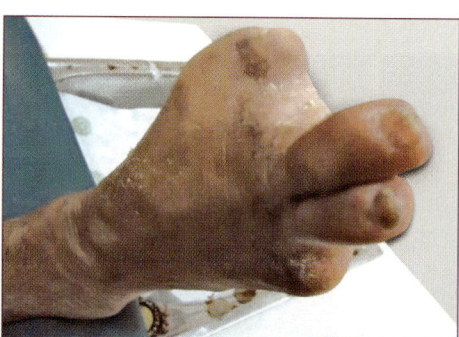

FIG. 10: Healing after amputation.

> **Take Home Messages**
>
> The following key recommendations of International Working Group on Diabetic Foot (IWGDF) for the diagnosis and management of patients with diabetes and DFU is helpful:
> - All diabetics should be examined annually for presence of PAD with history taking and palpating the foot pulses being mandatory
> - In patients with diabetes having a foot ulcer and PAD, signs and symptoms are not enough to predict wound healing. One of the following tests is helpful: A skin perfusion pressure of ≥40 mm Hg, toe pressure of 30 mm Hg or a $TcPO_2$ level of ≥25 mm Hg increase chances of wound healing.
>
>   *Revascularization:* International Working Group on Diabetic Foot advices that patients with diabetes having PAD and DFI are at a higher risk of major limb amputation. These patients should also receive aggressive cardiovascular risk management including cessation of smoking
> - Vascular imaging and revascularization should be considered in all patients with diabetes and PAD if the ulcer does not improve after 6 weeks of optimal management
> - And finally these patients should be under lifelong surveillance.

SUGGESTED READING

1. Brownrigg JR, Hinchliffe RJ, Apelqvist J, et al. Performance of prognostic markers in the prediction of wound healing or amputation among patients with foot ulcers in diabetes: a systematic review. Diabetes Metab Res Rev. 2016;32(Suppl 1):128-35.
2. Bus SA, van Netten JJ, Lavery LM, et al. IWGDF Guidance on the Prevention of Foot Ulcers in At-Risk Patients with Diabetes. 2015. [online] Available from www.iwgdf.org/files/2015/website_prevention.pdf. [Last accessed May, 2019].
3. Hinchliffe RJ, Brownrigg JRW, Apelqvist J, et al. IWGDF Guidance on the Diagnosis, Prognosis and Management of Peripheral Artery Disease in Patients with Foot Ulcers in Diabetes. 2015. [online] Available from www.iwgdf.org/files/2015/website_pad.pdf. [Last accessed May, 2019].
4. Public Health Agency of Canada. Reducing the risk of type 2 diabetes and its complications. In: Diabetes in Canada: Facts and Figures from a Public Health Perspective. in: Diabetes in Canada: Facts and Figures from a Public Health Perspective. 2011. [online] Available from www.phac-aspc.gc.ca/cd-mc/publications/diabetes-diabete/facts-figures-faitschiffres-2011/chap4-eng.php. [Last accessed May, 2019].
5. Registered Nurses' Association of Ontario (RNAO). Nursing Best Practice Guideline: Assessment and Management of Foot Ulcers for People with Diabetes. Toronto, ON: RNAO, 2005.

CASE 4: A Case of Diabetic Foot Infection

Ghanshyam Goyal

CASE HISTORY

A 60-year-old male, having type 2 diabetes mellitus (T2DM) for 10 years presented for the first time in the diabetic foot clinic with extensive gangrene of whole of left foot with involvement of lower one-third of leg (Figs. 1 and 2). Foul smell was emanating from the wound.

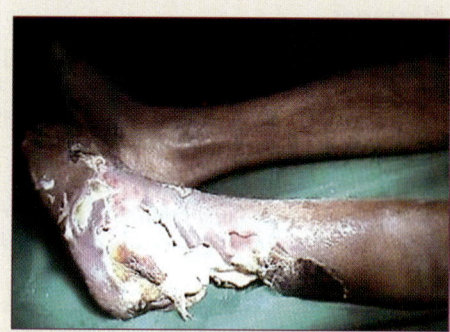
FIG. 1: At presentation.

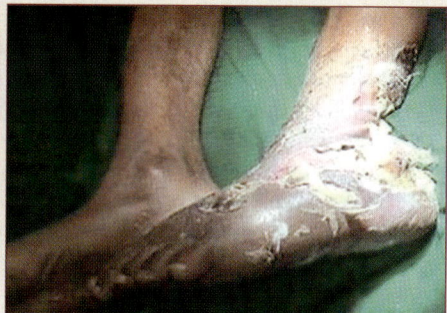
FIG. 2: At presentation.

DISCUSSION

Diabetic foot infections remain the most frequent complication of diabetes requiring hospitalization and are the most common precipitating events for lower leg amputation. Peripheral pulses, dorsalis pedis, posterior tibialis and popliteal were palpable in both feet.

In this patient extensive gangrene and destruction of whole of left foot with extension in lower one-third was present (the patient presented to us at a very late stage). It was a neuropathic foot with severe diabetic foot infection (DFI).

Diabetic foot infection is the most frequent complication of diabetes requiring admission and is also the most common factor leading to lower limb amputations. Any injury to the insensate foot like thermal injury, pressure or friction injury can go unnoticed and lead to infection. Factors that increase the risk of DFI are:
- Nonhealing ulcers of more than 1 month duration
- Recurrent foot ulcers
- Peripheral artery disease (PAD)
- Peripheral neuropathy (PN)
- Diabetic kidney disease
- History of barefoot walking.

Both Infectious Disease Society of America (IDSA) and International Working Group on the Diabetic Foot (IWGDF) state that the diagnosis and classification of infection is based on clinical signs and symptoms. In people with diabetes, inflammatory signs of infection may be masked due to PN and PAD. The severity of the infection should be judged based on the extent, depth and presence of systemic findings.

Clinical signs and symptoms of infection were evident in this patient's wound. His total WBC count was 18,000 cells/mm^3, hemoglbin 7.0 g/dL and serum creatinine was 2.9 mg/dL. His total protein was 5.4 and albumin 2.0. The patient was admitted and IV antibiotics—meropenem and linezolid along with insulin and other supportive medicines started. The patient was also given albumin and metabolically stabilized. Three units of blood was also transfused. The need for below knee amputations was discussed with family members and patient as it was a life-threatening situation.

Diabetic foot osteomyelitis (DFO) can occur in up to 60% of hospitalized patients and up to 20% of OPD patients. Osteomyelitis should be suspected when ulcers are present over bony prominences and fail to heal after adequate offloading or have associated soft

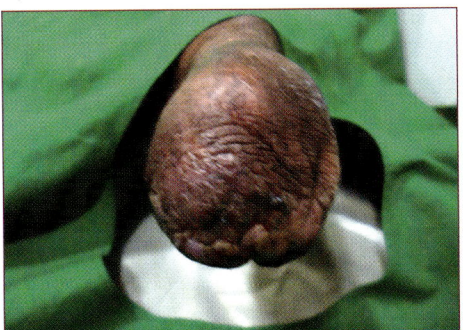 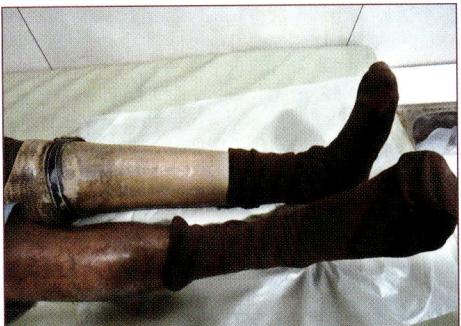

FIG. 3: Postamputation healed stump.   **FIG. 4:** Patient with below knee prosthesis.

tissue induration (sausage toe appearance). Probe-to-bone test is useful in diagnosing osteomyelitis. In most cases plain radiograph is adequate to evaluate and confirm DFO. MRI is considered the gold standard in diagnosis of DFO. When MRI is contraindicated or not available then CT scan can be considered.

History revealed that our patient was a heavy smoker (15–20 cigarettes/day).

Smoking cessation should be encouraged in all patients with diabetes, particularly in patients with diabetic foot.

The patient became critically ill and total WBC count had risen to 22,400 cells/mm^3. Urgent surgical consultation was done as infection was not only limb threatening but also life-threatening. After discussion with the patient and family members about the treatment modality and patient condition, it was decided to go for below knee amputation to save the life of the patient.

Lower limb amputations: One of the most challenging and difficult situation faced by clinicians, patients and family members is the decision to amputate or save the limb and it should always be decided on a case-to-case basis. The decision should be based on the patient's physical, mental and socioeconomic status. Amputations should always be the last resort when all efforts of limb salvage have failed.

Six weeks post below knee amputation (Fig. 3), our patient was provided with a below knee prosthesis (Fig. 4).

Take Home Message

- *Below knee amputation (BKA) is a life-changing event. It is the last resort when all options of saving the limb have failed. Sometimes BKAs are performed in order to save the life of the patient. Advances in surgical procedures and improved and advanced prosthesis have enabled patients to return to almost near normal life postamputation.*

SUGGESTED READING

1. Butalia S, Palda VA, Sargeant RJ, et al. Does this patient with diabetes have osteomyelitis of the lower extremity? JAMA. 2008;299(7):806-13.
2. Canadian Diabetes Association. (2006). Diabetes Statistics in Canada. [online] Available from www.diabetes.ca/how-you-can-help/advocate/why-federal-leadership-is-essential/diabetesstatistics-in-canada. [Last accessed June, 2019].
3. Dinh MT, Abad CL, Safdar N. Diagnostic accuracy of the physical examination and imaging tests for osteomyelitis underlying diabetic foot ulcers: Meta-analysis. Clin Infect Dis. 2008;47(4):519-27.

4. Doughty DB, Sparks B. Wound-healing physiology and factors that affect the repair process. In: Bryant RA, Nix DP (eds). Acute and Chronic Wounds: Current Management Concepts. St Louis, Missouri: Elsevier; 2016. pp. 63-81.
5. Lipsky BA, Aragón-Sánchez J, Diggle M, et al. IWGDF guidance on the diagnosis and management of foot infections in persons with diabetes. Diabetes Metabol Res Rev. 2016;32:45-74.
6. Lipsky BA, Berendt AR, Cornia PB, et al. 2012 Infectious Diseases Society of America clinical practice guideline for the diagnosis and treatment of diabetic foot infections. Clin Infect Dis. 2012;54(12):e132-73.
7. Lipsky BA. Bone of contention: Diagnosing diabetic foot osteomyelitis. Clin Infect Dis. 2008;47:528-30.

CASE 5 — A Case of Neuropathic Diabetic Foot
Ghanshyam Goyal

CASE HISTORY

A 57-year-old female having type 2 diabetes mellitus (T2DM) presented to the diabetic foot clinic with multiple ulcers on plantar surface of both feet (Figs. 1A and B).

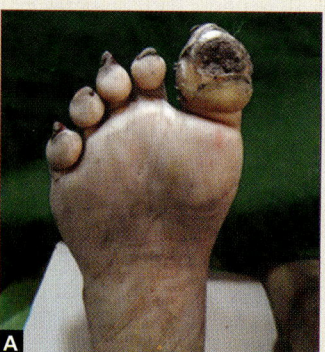 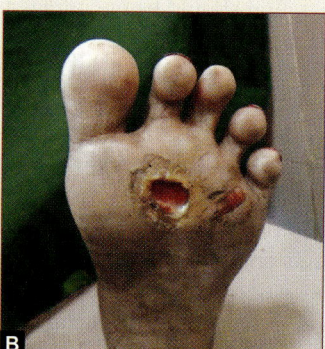

FIGS. 1A AND B: Ulcers at presentation.

DISCUSSION

Case History and Management

Risk of foot ulceration in patient with diabetes increases in presence of neuropathy, peripheral artery disease, previous ulceration or amputation, structural deformity, and high HbA1c.

Patient had a history of walking bare foot to the temple every morning. She had developed blisters and now the ulcers were nonhealing since last 5 months.

Although the prevalence and spectrum of foot problems varies in different regions of the world, the pathways to ulceration are probably very similar in most patients. Diabetic foot lesions frequently result from a patient simultaneously having two or more risk factors, with diabetic peripheral neuropathy playing a central role. This neuropathy leads to an insensitive and sometimes deformed foot, often causing an abnormal walking pattern. In people with neuropathy, minor trauma (e.g. from ill-fitting shoes, walking barefoot or an acute injury) can precipitate ulceration of the foot.

On examination, foot pulses, both dorsalis pedis and posterior tibial were palpable in both feet. Ankle/brachial index was normal. Neuropathic assessment was done, using a biothesiometer, and was found to be severely impaired in both feet. X-ray of both feet was normal. X-ray of foot is mandatory in all diabetic foot cases to exclude osteomyelitis.

The most common bedside tools to assess peripheral neuropathy (PN) are 10 g Semmes-Weinstein monofilament test (Fig. 2) and standard 128 Hz tuning fork. Quantitative assessment of PN is done using a biothesiometer (Fig. 3). A reading of more than 25 volts is indicative of high risk of future ulceration.

So this patient had nonhealing neuropathic ulcers in insensate feet caused by thermal injury and maybe minor trauma due to barefoot walking.

Debridement of ulcer was done in outpatient setting (Figs. 4 and 5). After debridement, the patient was put on a modified posterior slab (is an easy-to-use, preassembled synthetic splinting system). Made from polyurethane-coated fiberglass covered by polypropylene padding, which provides stabilization in 2–4 minutes and enables weight bearing in just 20 minutes in right foot and S K Offloading (a square piece of foam is rolled and placed below the ulcer and secured with micropore tape) in the left foot (Figs. 6 and 7).

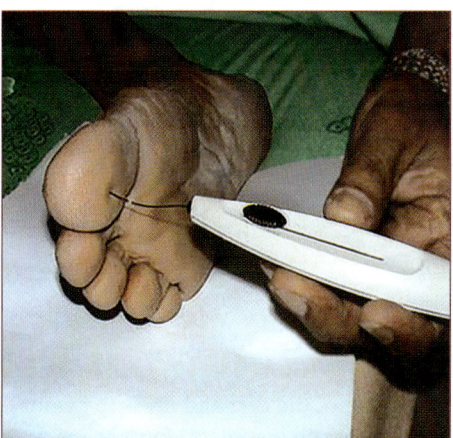

FIG. 2: Monofilament test.

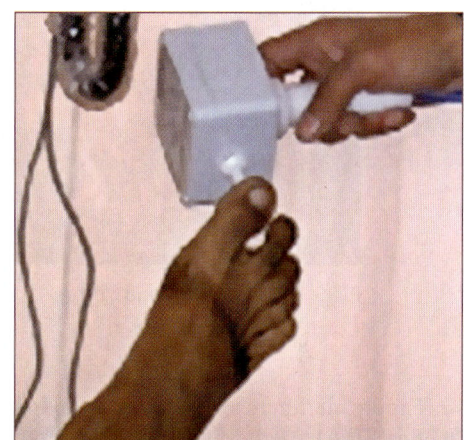

FIG. 3: Biothesiometer (VPT).

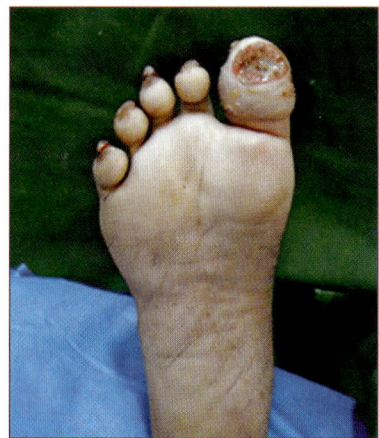

FIG. 4: Post debridement.

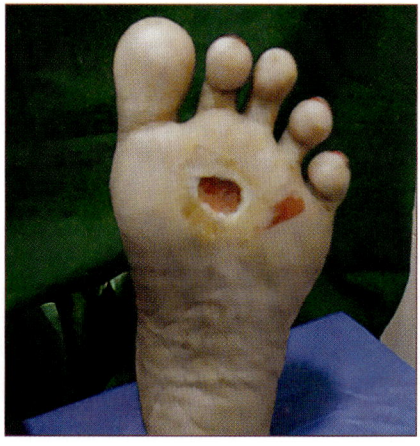

FIG. 5: Post debridement.

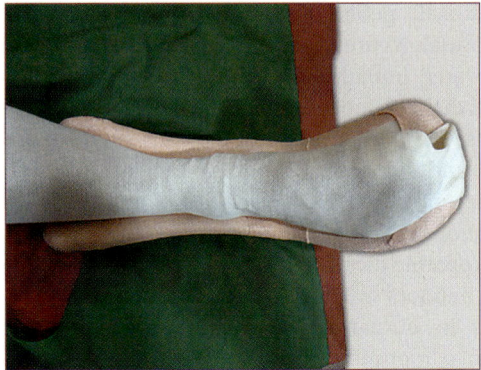

FIG. 6: Posterior slab.

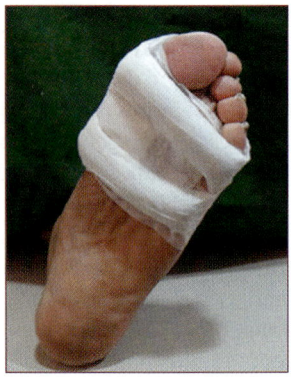

FIG. 7: S K offloading.

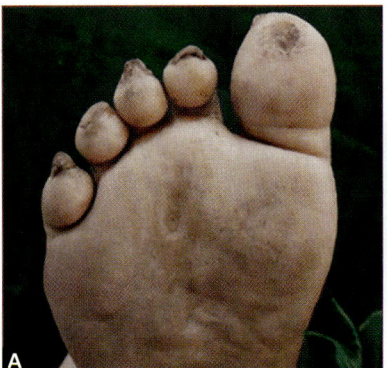

FIGS. 8A AND B: Wound closure.

Family members were trained as to how to take care of the cast and dress the wound at home. The patient was followed up after every 2 weeks and complete wound closure in both feet was achieved in 15 weeks (Figs. 8A and B).

Take Home Messages

Three basic tenets of management of any diabetic foot ulcer which should be addressed are:
- *Adequate debridement and infection control*
- *Adequate vascularity*
- *Adequate offloading.*

All people with diabetes should have their feet examined at least once a year to identify those at risk for foot ulceration.

The absence of symptoms in a person with diabetes does not exclude foot disorders; they may have asymptomatic neuropathy, peripheral artery disease, preulcerative signs or even an ulcer. The clinician should examine the feet with the patient both lying down and standing up, and should also inspect their shoes and socks.

Footcare education should be imparted to the patient and family members which should include:

- *A daily foot inspection, including areas between the toes*
- *Notify the appropriate healthcare provider at once if foot temperature is markedly increased, or if a blister, cut, scratch or ulcer has developed*
- *If the patient is having loss of protective sensation (LOPS) avoid walking barefoot, whether at home or outside. In this case study, the patient was walking barefoot to the temple as it was a cultural compulsion for her. We made her understand the sufferings that she and her family members underwent as a consequence of her walking barefoot and hopefully we were able to convince her not to do so in future.*

SUGGESTED READING

1. Craig AB, Strauss MB, Daniller A, et al. Foot Sensation Testing in the Patient With Diabetes: Introduction of the Quick & Easy Assessment Tool. Wounds. 2014;26(8):221-31.
2. Schaper NC, Van Netten JJ, Apelqvist J, et al. Prevention and management of foot problems in diabetes: a Summary Guidance for daily practice 2015, based on the IWGDF Guidance documents. Diabetes Metab Res Rev. 2016;32(Suppl 1):7-15.

SECTION 6

Genetics

CASE 1: Turner Syndrome with Hyperthyroidism
Anirban Mazumdar

CASE HISTORY

A 26-year-old female, amenorrheic for the past 2 years, presented with weight loss, palpitation, heat intolerance, increased appetite, and enlarging eyeballs for the past 3 months. Her menarche was at the age of 14 years and was irregular with delayed cycles from the very beginning. She was repeatedly prescribed hormone pills to regularize her cycle but this provided only temporary improvement. She was the only child of healthy unrelated parents of normal stature, father 165 cm and mother 155 cm. The family history was unremarkable.

On examination, she was short (133 cm), 37 kg in weight, normal 126/70 mm Hg blood pressure, poorly developed Tanner stage 2 breasts, high arched palate, broad chest, prominent eyes, low-set ears, webbed neck, low hairline, upward pointing fingernails and toenails (Fig. 1). The thyroid gland was soft and diffusely enlarged (Grade 3) without any bruit (Fig. 1). Eye examination revealed exophthalmos of moderate degree, mild congestion, normal eyeball movements and normal vision.

Antithyroid peroxidase antibody and TSH receptor antibody (TRAb) were strongly positive. Table 1 shows the results of laboratory investigations. Ultrasound (USG) of thyroid gland revealed diffused enlargement. There were no abnormalities in

TABLE 1: Laboratory evaluation.

Tests	Value	Normal range
Fasting plasma glucose	95 mg/dL	70–99
Serum creatinine	0.7 mg/dL	0.6–1.2
Prolactin	8.60 ng/mL	4–30
Follicle-stimulating hormone	35.36 mIU/mL	2–12
Luteinizing hormone	12.52 mIU/mL	1–18
Thyroid function tests		
Free T3	1,176 pg/dL	260–480
Free T4	3.20 ng/dL	0.85–1.80
Thyroid-stimulating hormone	0.007 µU/mL	0.50–5.50

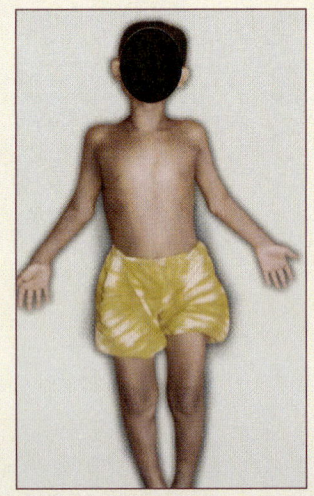

FIG. 1: Turner syndrome with increased carrying angles.

the chest X-ray and electrocardiography. USG of abdomen showed hypoplastic uterus, normal ovarian size and horseshoe kidneys. Chromosomal analysis of peripheral blood lymphocytes showed complete deletion of the short arm of second X chromosome. These results were compatible with a diagnosis of Graves' disease (GD) in Turner syndrome (TS). She was treated with methimazole and the hyperthyroid state resolved in 6 months. The changes in body weight and thyroid function were as below (Table 2).

On follow-up, her antithyroid medication was tapered down in next 3 months and she remained euthyroid thereafter. Estrogen replacement therapy was slowly started after the euthyroid state was maintained for 3 more months.

TABLE 2: Changes in body weight and thyroid function in 9 month follow-up.

	1st visit	3 months	6 months	9 months
Weight	37	43.5	49	47.1
FT3 (pg/dL)	1176	450	308	319
FT4 (ng/dL)	3.20	1.90	1.01	0.92
TSH (µU/mL)	0.007	0.5	5.02	9.90

(FT3: free triiodothyronine; FT4: free thyroxine; TSH: thyroid-stimulating hormone)

DISCUSSION

Turner syndrome is associated with increased prevalence of thyroid autoimmunity. Thyroid autoantibodies usually do not appear before the age of 8 years. The risk of developing subclinical or clinical thyroid dysfunction is greatest between 12 years and 14 years of age. Hashimoto thyroiditis is the most common thyroid dysfunction and GD has been reported rarely in TS. Thyroid autoantibodies are present in more than 60%, overt hypothyroidism in 24% and hyperthyroidism in 2.5% of TS. Hence, it is important to monitor thyroid and/or autoimmune markers of thyroid in patients with TS. GD occurs in all forms of chromosomal abnormalities associated with TS (45 XO or part deletion of X chromosome or mosaicism). However, the prevalence of thyroid abnormalities is not related to the type or severity of karyotype abnormality. Development of autoimmunity in TS is a complex interplay of genetic and environmental factors. T cells become autoreactive possibly due to haploinsufficiency of genes on the X chromosome. Apart from autoimmune thyroid disorders, many other autoimmune diseases like celiac disease, ulcerative colitis, Crohn's disease, psoriasis, idiopathic thrombocytopenic purpura, vitiligo and juvenile rheumatoid arthritis are commonly associated with TS.

Hyperthyroidism in patients with TS leads to acceleration of height velocity but our patient at 26 years age already reached her final adult height and hence did not gain further height. Estrogen has a great influence on thyroid economy as evidenced by the fact that thyroid diseases are more common among women, particularly during puberty and menopause. Estrogen increases thyroxin-binding globulin making the monitoring of GD difficult and possibly triggers thyroid autoimmunity. However, estrogen has both immunostimulating and immunosuppressive properties. Recently, the mechanism promoting T-cell activation and proliferation by estrogen has been elucidated. Because of this complex interplay between estrogen and thyroid disorders, the patient was treated with estrogen replacement therapy only after achievement of euthyroid status.

Relapse of hyperthyroidism after withdrawal of therapy is a common consequence and repeated course of antithyroid drug treatment may be required in future.

> **Take Home Message**
> - Importance of detecting coexisting autoimmune thyroid disease in patient with TS.

SUGGESTED READING

1. Livadas S, Xekouki P, Fouka F, et al. Prevalence of thyroid dysfunction in Turner's syndrome: a long-term follow-up study and brief literature review. Thyroid. 2005;15(9):1061-6.
2. Mohammad I, Starskaia I, Nagy T, et al. Estrogen receptor α contributes to T cell-mediated autoimmune inflammation by promoting T cell activation and proliferation. Sci Signal. 2018;11(526): eaap9415.
3. The Turner Syndrome Society of Canada. Turner Syndrome: Across the Lifespan. A guideline of the Turner Syndrome Study Group. Available from www.turnersyndrome.ca. [Last Accessed May 2019].

CASE 2: Hypogonadal Man with Leg Ulcers

Anirban Mazumdar

CASE HISTORY

A 58-year-old man was referred to our endocrine clinic for evaluation of long-standing erectile dysfunction which had not been previously investigated. He had left-sided leg ulcers unresponsive to numerous topical wound care therapies for 1 year. He was married for 20 years, had no children and was treated with intermittent intramuscular testosterone therapy for erectile dysfunction. He denied tobacco abuse. His intelligence was normal and he had a small business which he had been running successfully for the past 30 years.

Physical examination revealed a tall (174 cm) and overweight (BMI 28) man with long arms and legs. He had almost absent hair on the face, axilla, pubic area, and body (Fig. 1). He had bilateral gynecomastia (Fig. 2), micropenis, and small testes. Systemic examination was within normal limits. There were two deep skin ulcers on the left leg with raised irregular dark hyperkeratotic borders and necrotic base accompanied by mild pitting edema and appeared to be chronic venous ulcers (Fig. 3). The ulcers were

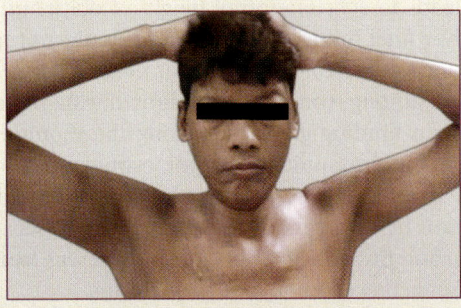

FIG. 1: Absent hair on the face, axilla and body.

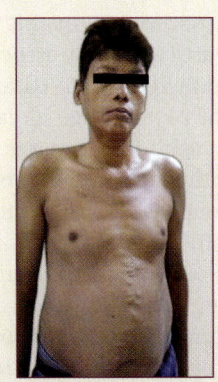

FIG. 2: Bilateral gynecomastia.

nonindurated and not fixed to deeper structures. Varicose veins were present on both legs. Dorsalis pedis pulses were palpable bilaterally and were normal.

Laboratory investigations revealed low hemoglobin (11.2 g/dL), with mild hypochromia and anisocytosis. Blood chemistry values were normal for renal function, liver function, and thyroid function tests. Endocrinological work-up revealed luteinizing hormone (LH) of 24 mIU/mL (normal range 0.8–6 mIU/mL), follicle-stimulating hormone (FSH) of 49.7 mIU/mL (normal range 1–11 mIU/mL), testosterone of 34 ng/dL (normal range 300–800 ng/dL), and bioavailable testosterone of 0.02 ng/mL (normal range for adult men >0.6 ng/mL). These results indicate a diagnosis of hypergonadotropic hypogonadism. Chromosomal analysis revealed a 47,XXY/46,XY karyotype which is typical for mosaic Klinefelter syndrome (KS). Arterial and venous Doppler of the legs did not show any evidence of deep venous thrombosis and an echocardiogram did not show any organic cardiac lesions. He was also tested for antinuclear antibody, rheumatoid factor and anticardiolipin IgM antibody, VDRL, hepatitis C antibodies, hepatitis B surface antigen, and human immunodeficiency virus, and all tests were negative.

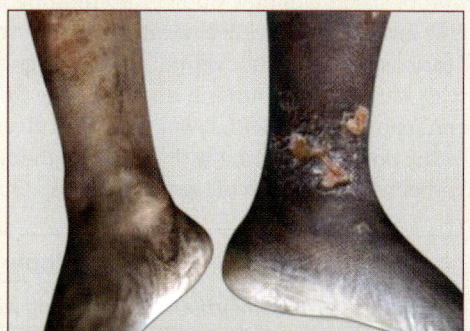

FIG. 3: Deep skin ulcers on the left leg.

Injectable androgen replacement therapy was started along with local conservative wound care treatment. His repeat total testosterone was 491 ng/dL, with improvement in FSH (10.6 mIU/mL) and LH (16.6 mIU/mL) level in 6 months. He also noticed progressive healing of his leg ulcers within 6 months of treatment with androgen.

DISCUSSION

Klinefelter's syndrome, first described in 1942 by Harry F Klinefelter, is a common cause of primary hypogonadism and erectile dysfunction in adult men. In this disorder, nondisjunction of the X chromosomes of either parent during meiotic division results in at least one extra X chromosome in the karyotype. This additional extra X chromosome results in the variable cognitive and physical abnormalities as seen in this syndrome and these abnormalities increase with the addition of each further supernumerary X chromosome. Gonadal consequences of the syndrome include small, firm testes, reduced sperm count and infertility. Hormonally, the KS patients have low testosterone levels because of testicular dysgenesis which leads to scant facial, sexual and body hair. Delayed fusion of the epiphyses of long bones due to subnormal sex hormone results in increased length of legs and consequently increase in height. KS can affect intellectual development also, leading to difficulty in social interactions. However, the mental capacity and the intelligence quotient score is not affected in mosaic KS as in our case.

Lower extremity ulceration is a recognized complication of KS, the pathogenesis of which is unclear. Chronic venous insufficiency, obesity, arterial dysplasia in lower limbs, and elevated plasminogen activator inhibitor-1 (PAI-1) leading to decrease in fibrinolysis are all implicated as possible etiologies of lower extremity ulcers in KS patients. This patient had normal arterial supply in lower limbs without any evidence of deep venous thrombosis on Doppler study. Autoimmune work-up was also negative. The appearance of his lower extremity ulcers was consistent with chronic venous ulcers and the presence of varicose veins further supported the diagnosis. Associations with metabolic syndrome, breast cancer, autoimmune diseases (like SLE), and thromboembolic diseases have all been reported in KS with lower extremity ulceration.

The positive outcome with androgen therapy in our case was consistent with that seen in other reported cases of leg ulcers in KS.

Take Home Message
- Consider KS in an infertile man presenting with lower extremity ulcers.

SUGGESTED READING

1. Igawa K, Nishioka K. Leg ulcer in Klinefelter's syndrome. J Eur Acad Dermatol Venereol. 2003;17(1): 62-4.
2. Radicioni AF, Ferlin A, Balercia G, et al. Consensus statement on diagnosis and clinical management of Klinefelter syndrome. J Endocrinol Invest. 2010;33(11):839-50.

CASE 3: An Obese Hyperactive Child
Anirban Mazumdar

CASE HISTORY

A 10-year-old, hyperactive, mild mentally retarded, obese boy was presented with undescended testes. He was second of two siblings and was born with birth weight 2.1 kg by cesarean section from nonconsanguineous parents. His mother was diabetic at 7 month of pregnancy and was treated with insulin. Knock knees were the first difficulty detected during walking when he was 2 years old. From two and half years of age, he was noted to have an insatiable appetite with subsequent obesity. Temper tantrums, impulsivity, aggression, and hyperactivity in new situations or in unfamiliar surroundings were noted from his early childhood. However, the vision and hearing development was normal.

Physical findings revealed a mentally retarded obese boy with bilateral undescended testes. His height was 120 cm (below 3rd centile) and body weight was 49 kg (above 97th centile). Eyes were almond shaped, upslanting with blue iris and with narrowing of temporal region on both side of face (Fig. 1). There was a markedly obese abdomen with striae over the flank, arm, and thigh. He had generalized lipomastia and small hands and feet. There was obvious evidence of

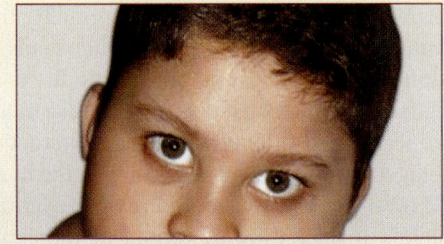

FIG. 1: PWS with distinctive facial features.

TABLE 1: Laboratory investigations.

Tests	Value	Normal range
Hemoglobin	11.8 g/dL	12–15
Fasting plasma glucose	79 mg/dL	70–99
Postprandial plasma glucose	148 mg/dL	70–140
Urea	14 mg/dL	4–29
Serum creatinine	0.6 mg/dL	0.5–1.4
Serum sodium	143 mEq/L	135–145
Serum potassium	4.9 mEq/L	3.5–5
Liver function tests	Normal	–
Thyroxine	8.39 µg/dL	4.0–12.3
Thyroid-stimulating hormone	2.0 µU/mL	0.4–4.8
Cholesterol	160 mg/dL	120–200
Triglycerides	248 mg/dL	54–110
High-density lipoprotein	36 mg/dL	35–80
Low-density lipoprotein	89 mg/dL	80–130

incomplete sexual development with bilateral undescended testes and small phallus (measuring 4 cm in length) which was buried in the suprapubic fat pad. Table 1 shows the results of the laboratory investigations.

In view of obesity and abdominal striae, morning (8 AM) basal cortisol was measured and was reported high. Overnight dexamethasone suppression test adequately suppressed cortisol (<1.10 µg/dL) and ruled out the possibility of hypercortisolism (Table 2).

TABLE 2: Evaluation of adrenal function.

Tests	Value	Normal range
Cortisol (8 AM)	32	5–25 µg/dL
Overnight 1 mg Dexa suppression	<1.10	<1.8 µg/dL

Ultrasound abdomen failed to detect enlarged adrenal glands and any sonological evidence of testicular tissue in the bilateral inguinal region or abdominal cavity. History and physical examination led to the diagnosis of Prader-Willi syndrome (PWS) which was confirmed by karyotyping (microdeletion of chromosome 15).

Both the testes remained impalpable and testosterone level failed to rise following 1 month of luteinizing hormone (LH) hormone therapy (1,000 IU thrice weekly). A futile endeavor with MRI abdomen to localize testes was made and surgical option for localization and removal of testes was not convincing to the pediatric surgeon.

In the absence of any definitive and effective treatment method for PWS, an attempt was made to manage the patient with lifestyle therapy. But progressive gain in weight remained unaltered even after cognitive behavioral therapy from psychiatry clinic. 3 years after his diagnosis, at the age of 13, he developed diabetes mellitus (Table 3). By this time, he gained in height from 120 to 145 cm (at 10th centile), gained in weight

TABLE 3: Laboratory evaluation on follow-up.

Tests	Value	Normal range
Fasting plasma glucose	277 mg/dL	70–99
Postprandial plasma glucose	396 mg/dL	70–140
Glycosylated hemoglobin	9.9%	4–5.6
Cholesterol	240 mg/dL	120–200
Triglycerides	373 mg/dL	54–110
High-density lipoprotein	54 mg/dL	35–80
Low-density lipoprotein	136 mg/dL	80–130
Free thyroxine	1.30 ng/dL	0.9–1.6
Thyroid-stimulating hormone	3.25 µU/mL	0.4–4.8

from 49 to 73 kg (at 97th centile) and BMI increased from 34 to 34.7. He was in a poor glycemic state with the following laboratory findings:

Glimepiride and metformin was started and he responded well with oral antidiabetic agents. Lifestyle and cognitive behavioral therapy continued to keep his body weight under control.

DISCUSSION

In 1956, Prader et al. reported a series of patients with Prader-Willi phenotypes and later deletions located between bands 15q11 and 15q13 were established as the cause for this syndrome. The estimated worldwide prevalence rate of this disorder is 1 per 45,000 population.

Most children present with symptoms of mental retardation and hyperphagia with progressive development of obesity. Intense craving for food leads to uncontrollable weight gain and morbid obesity. Muscle hypotonia, short stature, and hypogonadism are other characteristics of this syndrome. The diagnosis is based entirely on clinical observation. The patient, we have described, was presented with symptoms of hyperphagia, temper tantrums, obesity, delayed puberty, mild mental retardation and bilateral undescended testes. His diagnosis was confirmed by karyotyping (microdeletion of chromosome 15). He developed type 2 diabetes mellitus on follow-up at 13 years of age, like many other children with this syndrome.

Short stature is common in PWS and is mostly due to growth hormone deficiency. Our subject was short at presentation but maintained linear growth velocity and attained normal height on follow-up. The gain in height over 3 years had pushed his height from 3rd centile at 10 years of age to 10th centile at 13 years of age and hence growth hormone evaluation was not done.

Hypogonadism is also a very common feature of PWS due to both hypothalamic and testicular abnormalities. Cryptorchidism, the commonest testicular abnormality, is observed in approximately two-thirds of boys. Pubic and axillary hair may grow prematurely in children with PWS, but other features of puberty are generally delayed or incomplete. Bilateral cryptorchidism was present in our patient and we failed to locate intra-abdominal testes despite our best effort and he did not show any signs of puberty till 13 years of age.

Behavioral problems, like temper tantrums, stubbornness, and obsessive-compulsive behaviors compromising the academic performance are common features of PWS. Temper tantrums and stubbornness were very predominant behavioral issues of this child during presentation which improved over time, as did his academic performance.

Patients with PWS may develop central or obstructive sleep apnea (OSA). But this boy had no sleep-related symptoms, including consistent snoring, daytime sleepiness or long pauses in breathing (more than 5 s) and was not referred for a polysomnogram (sleep study).

Children and adolescents with PWS are at increased risk of glucose intolerance and diabetes especially who have a BMI above 95th percentile and/or taking growth hormone therapy due to concomitant growth hormone deficiency. Due to progressively increasing obesity (BMI 34.7, much above 95th percentile), the boy developed diabetes at the age of 13 years. Glycemic control was achieved with glimepiride and metformin along with lifestyle intervention. Therefore, obese children with behavioral problems should be evaluated for PWS. Not all PWS children are short and growth hormone deficient. Behavioral issues of these children may improve over time and type 2 diabetes mellitus (T2DM) is a common long-term sequelae which respond to oral antidiabetic agents.

> **Take Home Message**
> - *Consider PWS in obese children with behavioral problems.*

SUGGESTED READING

1. Donaldson MD, Chu CE, Cooke A, et al. The Prader-Willi syndrome. Arch Dis Child. 1994;70(1):58-63.
2. Ledbetter DH, Riccardi VM, Airhart SD, et al. Deletions of chromosome 15 as a cause of the Prader-Willi syndrome. N Engl J Med. 1981;304(6):325-9.
3. Lee PD. Endocrine and metabolic aspects of Prader-willi syndrome. In: Greenswag LR, Alexander RC (Eds). Management of Prader-willi Syndrome, 2nd edition. New York: Springer-Verlag; 1995. pp. 32-57.

CASE 4: A Boy with Macroorchidism
Anirban Mazumdar

CASE HISTORY

A 10-year-old boy was referred to the endocrine department for evaluation of hypothyroidism. The boy had behavioral disorder with autistic features and a thyroid-stimulating hormone (TSH) value of 5.8 mIU/mL. He was born to nonconsanguineous and healthy parents. Birth history revealed that he was delivered at term by lower segment cesarean section with a birth weight of 2.6 kg and developed neonatal jaundice, for which he was appropriately treated at neonatal intensive care for 10 days before being discharged from the hospital. He reached his developmental milestones on time until 8 years. As he grew older intellectual disability with poor attention and concentration, inadequate emotional responses, and mild social withdrawal became apparent. His elder brother was also suffering from mental retardation but no similar intellectual disability in any other member of his family was reported. His mother was healthy and exhibited normal intelligence.

General physical examination revealed an elongated face, prominent frontal bone, hypotonia, and hyperlaxity of the ligaments. The mouth had dental overcrowding and a high-arched palate. He had flat feet with plantar creases. His neurological and other system examinations were normal. His pubertal stage was Tanner stage 1 with absent axillary and pubic hair but he had bilaterally enlarged testis (macroorchidism) with 18 cc testicular volume as measured using Prader orchidometer beads (Fig. 1). He had no café-au-lait like skin lesions or any evidence of bony dysplasia of McCune-Albright syndrome. Repeat thyroid function test and thyroid peroxidase (TPO) antibody was normal. His follicle-stimulating hormone (FSH), luteinizing hormone (LH), and testosterone levels were in prepubertal range. Due to the presence of mental retardation and characteristic somatic features along with macroorchidism, a clinical diagnosis of Fragile X syndrome (FXS) was ascertained and karyotyping analysis confirmed the diagnosis (Table 1).

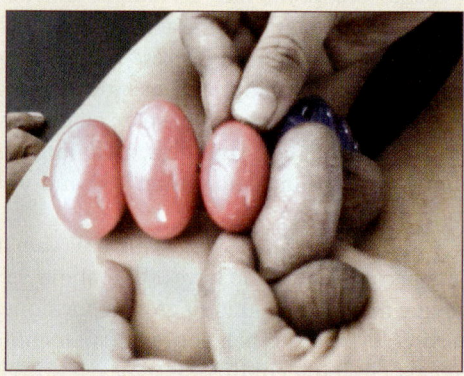

FIG. 1: Testicular volume (18 cc) measured using Prader orchidometer beads.

TABLE 1: Laboratory parameters.

Test	Value	Normal range
Fasting plasma glucose	82 mg/dL	70–99
Anti-thyroid peroxidase antibody	16 U/mL	<60
Free thyroxine	1.5 ng/dL	0.80–2.0
Thyroid-stimulating hormone	2.2 mIU/L	0.5–5.40
Follicle-stimulating hormone	2.5 IU/L	1–3 (prepubertal)
Luteinizing hormone	3.1 IU/L	0.3–6 (prepubertal)
Testosterone	78 ng/dL	300–1,100
Karyotyping	46,y, Fra (x)(q27-3) X chromosome showing fragile site (nonstaining gap on terminal end of long arm of X chromosome)	

DISCUSSION

Macroorchidism commonly occurs with FXS. Hypothyroidism, McCune-Albright syndrome, FSH-secreting pituitary macroadenoma or testicular neoplasm are other rare causes of macroorchidism. FXS is an X-linked disorder that may be diagnosed in both males and females. It is characterized by delayed physical and mental developmental milestones, learning disability, and dysmorphic features among children. The syndrome is usually not diagnosed until 8–9 years of age and on attaining puberty, the facial and body features of FXS become more evident. However, testicular enlargement or macroorchidism

TABLE 2: Clinical scoring for the seven most discriminant features of Fragile X syndrome.

Traits	Score
Skin soft and velvety on the palms with redundancy of skin on the dorsum of hand	2
Flat feet	2
Large and prominent ears	2
Plantar crease	1
Large testicles (postpubertal males only)	1
Familial history of intellectual disability	1
Autistic-like behavior	1
Total	10

is observed in 10–15% of all affected boys before puberty as in this case. A proposed clinical checklist and scoring is helpful for the clinical diagnosis for FXS (Table 2).

Patients with score higher than 5 have a significant yield of FXS and thus should be considered for testing to rule out the presence of the FXS. This 10-year-old boy displayed dysmorphic facial features, mental retardation, autistic behavior, macroorchidism, and history of intellectual disability of his elder brother. He did not have any clinical or biochemical features suggestive of hypothyroidism, McCune-Albright syndrome, FSH-secreting pituitary macroadenoma or testicular neoplasm. The presence of the many characteristic traits, mental retardation of unknown origin, and macroorchidism provided an initial clinical diagnostic clue.

Fragile X syndrome results from the mutation of the fragile X mental retardation 1 (*FMR1*) gene on the X chromosome (locus: Xq27.3). This abnormal gene, which can be passed from generation to generation, is usually inherited through the gene that is carried by women (X-linked dominant manner with reduced penetrance). Because the deleterious mutation is linked to the X chromosome, FXS is more frequent in males than in females. The chromosomal studies that identify the fragile site on the X chromosome (Xq27.3) can be a reliable diagnostic test for the detection of FXS. Confirmatory genetic tests (DNA analysis with southern blot and polymerase chain reaction) were not performed in our case due to the cost and its insignificant value in the further management of the boy.

Fragile X syndrome is the most common worldwide cause of inherited developmental disability. Because of a relatively high prevalence of FXS and its variable clinical phenotype, genetic test for FXS should be done in evaluation of all children with developmental delay. Early diagnosis allows the implementation of an appropriate therapeutic intervention program for children with FXS and genetic counseling for the family.

Take Home Message

- All boys and girls with mental retardation of unknown etiology should be tested for FXS regardless of family history.

SUGGESTED READING

1. Lubala TK, Lumaka A, Kanteng G, et al. Fragile X checklists: A meta-analysis and development of a simplified universal clinical checklist. Mol Genet Genomic Med. 2018;6(4):526-32.
2. Monaghan KG, Lyon E, Spector EB. Standards and Guidelines for fragile X testing: a revision to the disease-specific supplements to the Standards and Guidelines for Clinical Genetics Laboratories of the American College of Medical Genetics and Genomics. Genet Med. 2013;15(7):575-86.
3. Wattendorf DJ, Muenke M. Diagnosis and Management of Fragile X Syndrome. Am Fam Physician. 2005;72(1):111-3.

SECTION 7
Metabolism

CASE 1: Central Venous Sinus Thrombosis in a Type 2 Diabetes Mellitus Patient with Marked Hypertriglyceridemia

Debmalya Sanyal

CASE HISTORY

A 50-year-old Indian male known to have type 2 diabetes mellitus (T2DM) for 5 years presented with sudden onset diffuse headache accompanied. There was no focal neurodeficit. Computed tomography scan revealed intra cerebral hemorrhage. Magnetic resonance imaging of brain and magnetic resonance venogram showed hemorrhagic infarct with almost complete occlusion of superior sagittal sinus. (Fig. 1). Despite regular oral anti-diabetic medications (metformin 2g), his glycaemic control was not optimal with fasting plasma glucose of 234 mg/dL and postprandial plasma glucose of 321 mg/dL and HbA1c of 8.3%, but arterial pH, serum osmolality, bicarbonate and serum lipase were also within the normal ranges. His lipid profile revealed extremely high serum triglyceride level but total cholesterol, high-density lipoprotein, low-density lipoprotein cholesterol level, lipoprotein (a) were all within normal limits (Table 1). He had no family history of hypertriglyceridemia, no history of alcohol/beer intake, with normal coagulopathy screen. A diagnosis of superior sagittal sinus thrombosis in a case of uncontrolled diabetes and hypertriglyceridemia was made. The patient was treated with basal bolus insulin, heparin and was discharged on basal insulin and metformin along with warfarin, fenofibrate 200 mg, atorvastatin 40 mg.

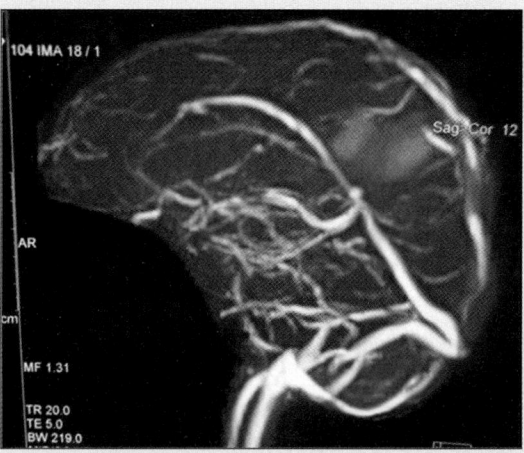

FIG. 1: Magnetic resonance imaging of brain and magnetic resonance venogram showing subacute hemorrhagic infarct in left parietal lobe with almost complete occlusion of superior sagittal sinus sparing only posterior aspect.

TABLE 1: Baseline laboratory examinations.

Test	Result	Normal
Triglyceride	2,578 mg/dL	<150
Low-density lipoprotein cholesterol	126 mg/dL	<100
High-density lipoprotein cholesterol	47 mg/dL	>40
Lipoprotein(a)	16	<30
Total leucocyte count	9,300 per mm^3	4,000–11,000
Arterial	7.42 pH	7.35–7.45
Serum osmolality	286 mosm/kg (mmol/kg)	275–295
Serum sodium	128 mEq/L	136–149
Bicarbonate	27 mEq/L	21–28
Serum lipase	30 U/L	<60
Polymorphonucleur neutrophil	72%	45–75%
Urea	24 mg/dL	21–43
Serum creatinine	0.9 mg/dL	<1.5
Serum amylase	55 U/L	<100

DISCUSSION

The association between diabetes and venous thromboembolism (VTE) is unclear. Diabetes may cause a hypercoagulable state with altered platelet function, coagulation and fibrinolytic systems. Diabetes with hyperketonaemia and hyperosmolarity may further increase thrombotic complications due to dehydration. There are previous case reports of central venous sinus thrombosis (CVST) in type 1 diabetes mellitus (T1DM) with diabetic ketoacidosis and dehydration or hyperosmolarity in association with T2DM. In our case the major risk factors for CVST are uncontrolled diabetes mellitus and extremely high triglyceridemia diabetes but in the absence of concomitant ketoacidosis, hyperosmolar state or any known prothrombotic conditions.

In the present case hypertriglyceridemia was one of the predisposing factors for developing CVST. Meta-analysis measuring the triglyceride levels to investigate its effect on VTE found higher triglyceride levels. In our case, uncontrolled hyperglycaemia and extremely high triglyceridemia may have increased our patient's thrombotic risk, even in the absence of dehydration or ketoacidosis.

Take Home Message

- Clinicians need to consider uncontrolled diabetes and hypertriglyceridemia as a predisposing factor for CVST, and need for active screening in patients with CSVT. Adequate preventive measures may be initiated in patients WITH uncontrolled diabetes and hypertriglyceridemia to prevent CSVT.

SUGGESTED READING

1. Ageno W, Becattini C, Brighton T, Selby R, Kamphuisen PW. Cardiovascular risk factors and venous thromboembolism: a meta-analysis. Circulation. 2008;117:93-102.
2. Keenan CR, Murin S, White RH. High risk for venous thromboembolism in diabetics with hyperosmolar state: Comparison with other acute medical illnesses. J Thromb Haemost. 2007;5:1185-90.
3. Usdan LS, Choong KWL, McDonnell ME. Type 2 diabetes mellitus manifesting with a cerebral vein thrombosis and ketoacidosis. Endocr Pract. 2007;13:687-90.

CASE 2: To be Taken with A Pinch of Salt

Kalyan Kumar Gangopadhyay

CASE HISTORY

A 22-year-old male was admitted with a history of collapse. He had been feeling unwell for a day or two with nonspecific symptoms of nausea, headache and dizziness. On admission, he was afebrile and was hemodynamically stable. However he was agitated with a Glasgow coma scale of 11/15. There were no focal neurological signs. CT head was unremarkable. His laboratory results revealed Na = 115 mmol/L, K = 1.5 mmol/L, serum creatinine = 1.31 mg/dL, random glucose = 164 mg/dL, cortisol = 37.3 µg/dL, urine osmolality = 241 mOsm/kg, urine sodium ≤10 mmol/L. There was no history of drug abuse or diuretic abuse. In the absence of any other cause, the collapse was attributed to hyponatremia. He was treated with 0.9% NaCl and made full recovery after 24 hours. However, further history available subsequently revealed that he had recently joined a building firm as a truck driver without any air-conditioning and spent a substantial amount of time lifting heavy materials. He reported that he had been sweating profusely, but at the same time had been drinking excessive amounts of water as suggested by various advertising campaigns to prevent dehydration during strenuous work in hot conditions.

DISCUSSION

Exercise-associated hyponatremia (EAH) is a well described entity, not just limited to athletes. This usually refers to an acute drop in blood sodium concentration (Na^+) during or immediately following physical activity. With rising global temperatures, it has now achieved an even greater significance.

Epidemiology of Exercise-associated Hyponatremia

The EAH was initially identified more than 30 years ago amongst endurance athletes. However, it was in early 2000, following the death of two otherwise healthy marathon runners, that this complication became known both to the lay public and the sports medicine community. In the past decade, several deaths have occurred amongst soldiers, policemen, footballers other than marathon runners. During routine screening for research purposes asymptomatic EAH has been found to be present in about a third of rugby players and marathon runners.

Pathogenesis

The EAH has multiple overlapping etiologies with complex pathogenesis which is highlighted in Flowchart 1. However the primary mechanism leading to EAH is the overconsumption of hypotonic fluids, usually in the face of excess sweating. Studies done in athletes reveal that the mean sweat Na^+ is around 40–50 mmol/L and the mean sweat rate is around 1–1.25 L/h, although there is some variation in both the sweat rate and sweat sodium concentration. Hence an athlete or a manual laborer working in hot conditions during the summer season may lose a considerable amount of sodium through sweating. On the other hand, the perils of dehydration have been so well publicized that some people drink excessive amounts of water/fluids to compensate for the fluid loss. The usual sports drinks have lower concentration of sodium as compared to sweat sodium (higher sodium in the drink may make them unpalatable). Hence loss of sodium followed by replacement with salt poor fluids might be one of the important factors in propagating the hyponatremia.

There may be other factors leading to the hyponatremia. Arginine vasopressin (AVP), which is usually suppressed in the presence of hypo-osmolality, may not be suppressed in some athletes. There are also several potential stimuli to AVP release including nonspecific stress, heat exposure, medication use [Nonsteroidal anti-inflammatory drugs (NSAID), selective serotonin reuptake inhibitors], interleukin 6, during exercise. Hence unsuppressed AVP and salt poor fluid intake, both together helps propagate the hyponatremia.

Another speculated mechanism is the inappropriate level of osmotically active sodium. As much as one-fourth of the total body sodium may exist in skin, bone and cartilage stores. These sodium stores are dynamic and may help reduce the risk of hyponatremia by exiting this pool. Hence, it has been hypothesized that athletes, who develop EAH, may fail to activate this pool of sodium but this mechanism remains speculative.

Some athletes may have a large volume of fluid in the stomach (from recent ingestion), and rapid absorption of this fluid after the athletic event (as gastrointestinal blood flow increases once exercise ceases) may contribute to the hyponatremia.

Treatment

The treatment should be directed towards managing the acute hyponatremia which is the hallmark of EAH. Central pontine myelinolysis, a complication of rapid treatment of chronic hyponatremia, is not applicable here as the onset of hyponatremia in EAH is less than 48 hours. The treatment should be guided by signs and symptoms as outlined

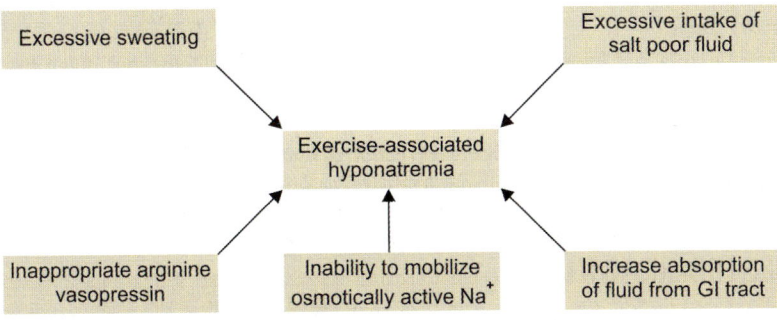

FLOWCHART 1: Suggested mechanisms leading to exercise-associated hyponatremia.

TABLE 1: Management of exercise-associated hyponatremia based on clinical symptoms and signs.

Symptoms and signs	Management
Nonspecific symptoms, dizziness, fatigue, nausea but fully conscious	Fluid restriction/oral hypertonic solutions
Altered mental function, confusion, headache, vomiting	Intravenous boluses of 100 mL 3% NaCl repeated till clinical improvement
Seizures, coma	Urgent intravenous 3% NaCl bolus repeated until clinical recovery

in Table 1. Encephalopathy associated with the hyponatremia should be treated with intravenous hypertonic saline, and till date, there have not been any cases of central pontine myelinolysis resulting from this. Isotonic saline has also been tried but the recovery is substantially delayed.

Prevention of Exercise-associated Hyponatremia

It is important to understand that most of the deaths associated with EAH could have been prevented with judicious use of fluid and salt. The existing myth that even when people do moderate levels of exercise, they must "drink as much as possible" may act as the starting point for EAH. The existing "rehydration drinks" available in the market all are hypotonic solutions and hence, taking large amounts of water/hypotonic fluids, over a short period of time may fuel the EAH. One may hypothesize that EAH is not just limited to athletes, but may happen in people who spend a substantial amount of time doing moderate laborious work under the sun in hot countries, like policemen, construction workers, farmers, etc. Hence the first advice should be "to drink according to your thirst".

While it seems to be logical to take sodium supplements to prevent EAH, the role of sodium supplementation remains controversial, with some studies showing attenuated fall in plasma sodium while others have not shown any difference. Hence the 3rd International Exercise Associated Hyponatremia Consensus Development Conference have suggested that while sodium ingestion during the periods of exercise may attenuate the fall in sodium concentration, it alone cannot prevent EAH if there is excessive fluid intake.

Take Home Messages

- Exercise-induced hyponatremia although well-known, is still an underdiagnosed entity and can be potentially fatal
- Excessive sweating (salt loss) followed by excessive water/salt poor fluid intake may be primary cause
- Exercise-associated hyponatremia may not be limited to athletes, but given the rise of temperature worldwide may be seen in individuals doing even moderately heavy work in the hot weather
- Treatment of EAH is directed at acute correction of hyponatremia
- Drinking according to thirst is the mainstay of prevention of EAH.

SUGGESTED READING

1. Hew-Butler T, Loi V, Pani A, et al. Exercise-associated Hyponatremia: 2017 Update. Front Med (Lausanne). 2017;4:21.

Section 7: Metabolism

CASE 3
Familial Partial Lipodystrophy Masquerading as Polycystic Ovarian Syndrome: Rare or Overlooked?

Subhankar Chowdhury, Partha Pratim Chakraborty

CASE HISTORY

Patient A

A 22-year-old lady born out of nonconsanguineous union presented to our endocrinology clinic with progressively increasing hair growth in a male pattern distribution for preceding 2 years associated with oligomenorrhea for last 7 years. She experienced menarche at the age of 12 years and had been managed with oral contraceptive pills with a diagnosis of polycystic ovarian syndrome (PCOS). Clinical examination revealed a lean individual with excess hair growth over face and body. A thorough evaluation also revealed marked loss of subcutaneous fat from her four limbs, buttocks and abdomen giving her a muscular appearance. However, subcutaneous fat in the face (Figs. 1A to C), palms and soles was preserved and she had no acanthosis or clitoromegaly.

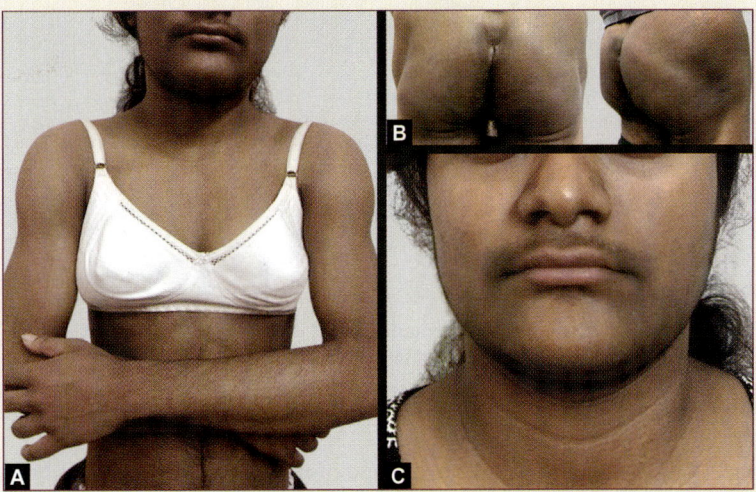

FIGS. 1A TO C: Loss of subcutaneous fat from upper limbs giving rise to a muscular appearance (A), loss of fat from buttocks (B) with preserved subcutaneous fat over face and neck (C); (Patient A).

Patient B

A 16-year-old girl having menarche at 10 years of age had presented to her gynecologist for oligomenorrhea since menarche and had been diagnosed with PCOS. She used to bleed after progesterone withdrawal. A thorough history revealed that loss of fat from

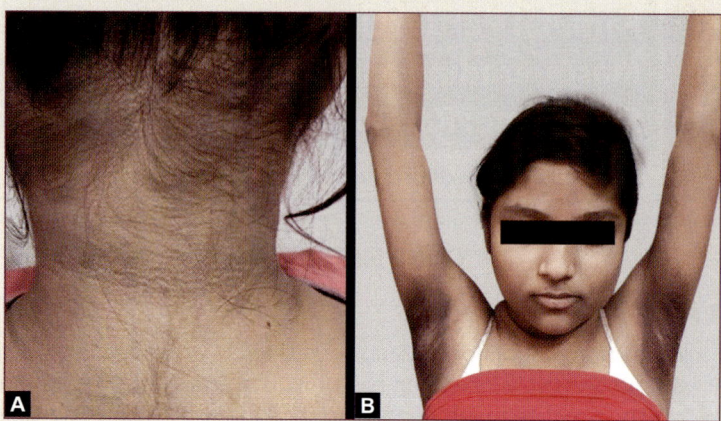

FIGS. 2A AND B: Acanthosis over nape of neck (A) and both axillae (B) (Patient B). There is no loss of subcutaneous fat from the face.

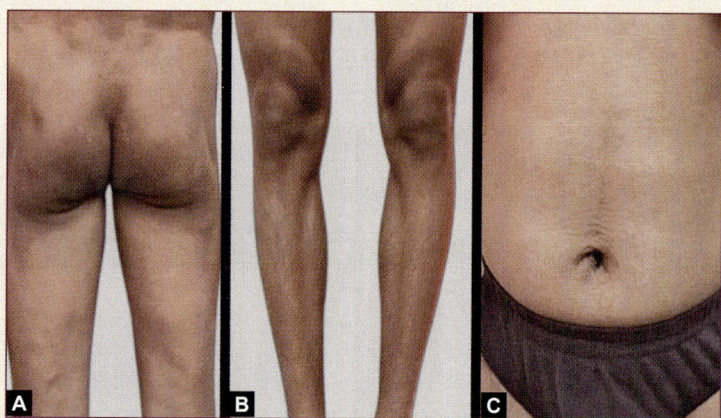

FIGS. 3A TO C: Reduced subcutaneous fat from buttocks (A) and lower extremities (B) with preservation of fat over abdomen (C); (Patient B).

the buttocks was noticed since early childhood which had not progressed significantly and the issue had been ignored.

Examination revealed acanthosis over nape of neck and both axillae. Subcutaneous fat was absent from her buttocks and lower limbs; however, her face, upper extremities and trunk were spared (Figs. 2 and 3). She had no hirsutism, hepatomegaly or clitoral enlargement.

Relevant investigations, done in these two ladies have been summarized in Table 1. Both of them were put on combination oral contraceptive (ethinyl estradiol and desogestrel) along with a detailed instruction about lifestyle modification that included dietary advice by a trained dietician and structured physical exercise. The first patient was also advised spironolactone and local cosmetic therapy for facial hirsutism. After 6 months of treatment she noticed significant decrease in facial hirsutism and spironolactone was withdrawn. Her serum testosterone after a year of presentation is 136 ng/dL.

TABLE 1: Summary of investigations.

Parameters (Normal range)	Patient A	Patient B
Fasting plasma glucose (70–100 mg/dL)	91	105
Plasma glucose at 2 h following 75 g of oral glucose (<140 mg/dL)	146	156
Fasting insulin (1.4–14 mIU/L)	19.6	26.9
Serum insulin at 2 h following 75 g of oral glucose (60–80 mIU/L)	>300	184
Serum glutamic-oxaloacetic transaminase (20–48 U/L)	48	32
Serum glutamic-pyruvic transaminase (10–40 U/L)	76	36
Triglyceride (<150 mg/dL)	168	121
High-density lipoprotein cholesterol (>50 mg/dL)	40	29
Uric acid (3.5–6.5 mg/dL)	5	6.2
Thyroid-stimulating hormone (0.5–5 mIU/L)	3.57	3.2
Prolactin (4–23 ng/mL)	15.5	7.9
Follicle-stimulating hormone (1–13 mIU/mL)	2.8	5.6
Luteinizing hormone (1–9 mIU/mL)	3.6	17.5
17-hydroxyprogesterone (17-OH-P) (<2 ng/mL)	3.8	1.9
17-OH-P 1 h after 250 µg of injection synthetic ACTH (<10 ng/mL rules out congenital adrenal hyperplasia)	5.3	Not done
Cortisol 1 h after 250 µg of injection synthetic ACTH (>18 µg/dL rules out adrenal insufficiency)	25.4	Not done
Testosterone (8–60 ng/dL)	224.6	84.1
Androstenedione (0.3–3.5 ng/dL)	5.5	2.9
Dehydroepiandrosterone sulfate (DHEAS) (35–430 µg/dL)	36.4	67
Ultrasonography abdomen	Fatty liver, enlarged ovaries (RO: 17.4 cc, LO: 15 cc) with multiple small follicles (4–7mm) in the periphery	Fatty liver, enlarged ovaries (RO: 12.8 cc, LO: 13 cc) with multiple small follicles (4–7 mm) in the periphery
CT scan of abdomen	Bulky ovaries	
Whole body fat by DEXA scan (Normal range in this age group taking into account sex and BMI is 25–35%)	14.4%	19.7%
Complete blood count, C3, C4, antinuclear factor, HIV serology, and urine examination for RBC and protein	Normal	Normal

(ACTH: adrenocorticotropic hormone; BMI: body mass index; CT: computed tomography; DEXA: dual energy X-ray absorptiometry; HIV: human immunodeficiecy virus; LO: left ovary; TSH: thyroid-stimulating hormone; RBC: red blood cells; RO: right ovary)

DISCUSSION

Lipodystrophy (LD) is a heterogeneous group of rare metabolic disorders associated with complete or partial lack of adipose tissue (lipoatrophy) in certain body areas in absence of nutritional deprivation or catabolic state, often accompanied with excess of adipose tissue (lipohypertrophy) elsewhere. Based on etiology and extent of loss of adipose tissue mass it can be subdivided into four major categories—(1) congenital generalized lipodystrophy (CGL), (2) familial partial lipodystrophy (FPLD), (3) acquired generalized lipodystrophy (AGL), and (4) acquired partial lipodystrophy (APL). Familial partial lipodystrophy (FPLD) is characterized by selective regional loss of fat affecting the limbs, buttocks and hips and is often associated with hypertrophy of adipose tissue in other areas. The inheritance could be autosomal recessive or autosomal dominant and a number of candidate genes have been identified.

The inherited forms could be face-sparing (Dunnigan variety) or could be restricted only to the extremities sparing both face and trunk (Köbberling type). Dunnigan variety, also known as type 2 FPLD, is characterized by loss of adipose tissue in the lower limbs and buttocks and, to a minor extent, in the abdominal subcutaneous fat depots with fat accumulations in the face, neck, axillae, labia and visceral adipose tissue and apparent muscular hypertrophy. Increased accumulation of subcutaneous fat in the face and neck has been reported in FPLD patients giving them a Cushingoid appearance. Loss of subcutaneous fat from the limbs results in a muscular appearance and poses difficulty in diagnosis in males and exercising females. Köbberling syndrome or the type 1 FPLD is clinically identified by loss of adipose tissue in the buttocks and limbs associated with an accumulation of fat in the trunk, particularly subcutaneous and visceral abdominal fat, and occasionally fat accumulations in the face and neck. Fat distribution in FPLD is typically normal in early childhood, with loss of fat occurring around puberty. The pattern of lack of subcutaneous fat points toward possible Dunnigan variety and Köbberling variety of FPLD in patient A and patient B respectively.

Differentiation of congenital form from acquired form of partial lipodystrophy becomes difficult at times as the acquired form also begins in childhood or adolescence and a detailed pedigree analysis may be helpful.

The most common etiology of oligo-/amenorrhea and hirsutism in young girls and premenopausal adult females is PCOS. Currently there are three definitions (National Institute of Health, Rotterdam, Androgen Excess PCOS Society) for PCOS that take into account clinical and/or biochemical hyperandrogenism, chronic oligo- or anovulation and ovarian morphology on ultrasound in varying combinations to make the diagnosis. However, all these criteria are consistent in that PCOS is a diagnosis of exclusion. The Endocrine society recommends that primary hypothyroidism, hyperprolactinemia and nonclassical congenital adrenal hyperplasia should be excluded in all patients with suspected PCOS and certain diagnoses should be considered in selected women depending on presentation. Syndromes of severe insulin resistance are considered a very rare disease simulating PCOS.

Polycystic ovarian syndrome is more frequent in partial lipodystrophy compared to nonlipodystrophic patients and infertility and abortion are more common in these patients. However, it is not clear why some patients with lipodystrophy develop secondary PCOS while others do not.

> **Take Home Messages**
>
> - *Polycystic ovarian syndrome is a diagnosis of exclusion and mere presence of clinical/biochemical hyperandrogenism, oligo-/amenorrhea and polycystic ovaries do not confirm PCOS*
> - *All the possible clinical conditions mimicking PCOS, regardless of their prevalence should be considered and excluded in appropriate patients, particularly in lean individuals with or without acanthosis nigricans*
> - *Increased awareness among all clinicians including gynecologists, physicians and general practitioners is needed about lipodystrophy and a thorough clinical examination is required in all such patients focusing on performing a muscle/fat distribution screen with appropriate consent and chaperoning to identify abnormal fat distribution.*

SUGGESTED READING

1. Brown RJ, Araujo-Vilar D, Cheung PT, et al. The Diagnosis and Management of Lipodystrophy Syndromes: A Multi-Society Practice Guideline. J Clin Endocrinol Metab. 2016; 101(12):4500-11.
2. Garg A. Lipodystrophies: Genetic and Acquired Body Fat Disorders. J Clin Endocrinol Metab. 2011;96(11):3313-25.
3. Legro RS, Arslanian SA, Ehrmann DA, et al. Diagnosis and Treatment of Polycystic Ovary Syndrome: An Endocrine Society Clinical Practice Guideline. J Clin Endocrinol Metab. 2013; 98(12):4565-92.

SECTION 8
Ovaries

CASE 1: Polycystic Ovarian Syndrome: A Common Problem

Rahin Mahata, Chandan Mishra, Partha Sarathi Choudhury, Anirban Sinha, Animesh Maiti, Asish Kumar Basu

CASE HISTORY

A 25-year-old married lady presented with primary infertility. She had menstrual irregularity in the form of oligomenorrhea since menarche (attained at 13 years of age) and hirsutism for the last 6 years. She was known hypothyroid for last 7 years and was on L-thyroxine (112.5 μg/day) maintaining euthyroidism. She was nondiabetic, nonhypertensive and was on intermittent OCP. Family history of diabetes was absent. Table 1 summarizes the baseline clinical parameters and the investigation done are presented in Table 2.

Diagnosis: Obese polycystic ovarian syndrome with type 2 diabetes mellitus (T2DM) and primary hypothyroidism.

TABLE 1: Clinical examination.

Parameters	Value
Pulse rate	78 beats/min
Blood pressure	110/70 mm Hg
Height	151.7 cm
Weight	66 kg
Body mass index (BMI)	28.67 kg/m^2 (obese Gr 1, Asian)
Waist circumference	101 cm
Hip circumference	106 cm
Waist hip ratio (WHR)	0.95

Masculine physique, temporal balding +, goiter grade I, acanthosis: grade 3, no acne, striae or bruise, moderate hirsutism + (FG score: 15/36), clitoromegaly + (clitoral index: 72 mm^2; abnormal >35 mm^2) (Figs. 1A and B). Rest of the systemic examination appeared normal.

TABLE 2: Investigation (on admission).

Parameters	Value
Fasting plasma glucose	178 mg/dL
Postprandial plasma glucose	298 mg/dL
FT4	1.44 ng/dL
Thyroid-stimulating hormone	2.91 microIU/mL
Total testosterone	174.7 ng/dL (normal <50 ng/dL)
Serum 17(OH) progesterone	1.8 ng/mL (normal <2 ng/mL)
Cortisol	14.9 µg/dL
Prolactin	5.32 ng/mL
Dehydroepiandrosterone sulfate	165 µg/dL (48–361 µg/dL)
Anti-Müllerian hormone	19.2 ng/mL
Follicle-stimulating hormone	4.98 mIU/ml
Luteinizing hormone	5.58 mIU/mL
USG of pelvis (TVS)	
Left ovary	19 cc (follicle no. <10)
Right ovary	21 cc (follicle no. >12)

Peripherally arranged follicles with echogenic stroma present; uterus: normal size. Endometrial thickness = 6 mm; no adnexal mass found.
USG abdomen: Grade I fatty liver, no adrenal SOL noted.

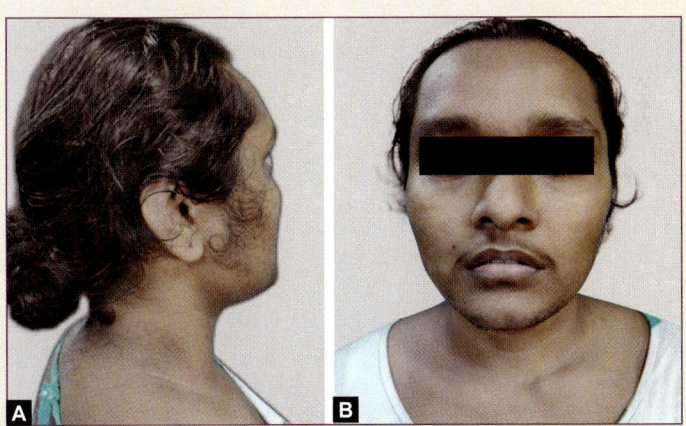

FIGS. 1A AND B: Acanthosis nigricans and hirsutism.

DISCUSSION

Polycystic ovarian syndrome is the most common endocrine disorder in reproductive age group with a prevalence of 5–10%. Among them, about two-thirds are insulin resistant. Impaired glucose tolerance (IGT) or frank diabetes is found in about 45% of PCOS women by their fourth decade.

Therefore, early screening and periodic monitoring of plasma glucose would be helpful to pick up a substantial number of cases of dysglycemia at the very beginning so as to initiate early intervention in these cases.

> **Take Home Message**
>
> - *As about two-thirds of patients with PCOS are insulin resistant, early screening and periodic monitoring of plasma glucose would be helpful to detect dysglycemia at the earliest.*

SUGGESTED READING

1. DeGroot's Text book of Endocrinology. 7th edition.
2. Fritz MA, Speroff L. Clinical gynecologic endocrinology and infertility. 8th edition. 2012.
3. Harrison's Text book of Internal Medicine. 19th edition. November 2014.
4. Melmed S, Polonsky KS, Larsen PR, Kronenberg HM. William's Text book of Endocrinology. 13th edition. January 2016.

SECTION 9

Pancreas

CASE 1: Hypoglycemia Workup
Binayak Sinha

CASE HISTORY

A 50-year-old physician was found unconscious in bed by his wife, one morning. He was taken into the emergency room nearby where his capillary blood glucose (CBG) was found to be 32 mg/dL. He was resuscitated with intravenous glucose. He had been previously fit and well with no significant ailments in the past and was on no medications. A nonsmoker, he used alcohol socially and had no significant family history. He was a slim gentleman with a body mass index (BMI) of 21 kg/m^2. He was hemodynamically stable and no abnormal signs were found. On workup, he showed a normal hematocrit and leukocyte count with normal renal and liver function. His serum electrolytes and thyroid function was normal. His ECG and chest X-ray were completely within normal limits. However on the ward the same day he was again found to be irritable and sweaty and a CBG showed 48 mg/dL. He was then referred to the endocrinologist.

The patient was found to be hypoglycemic again on admission with a CBG of 44 mg/dL. His serum cortisol was normal and no signs of sepsis or malignancy were found. When he was symptomatic with hypoglycemia his blood tests revealed a blood glucose of 37 mg/dL, serum insulin of 28 μu/mL, C-peptide 2.4 nmol/L and a serum proinsulin level of 8.3 pmol/L. Based on these we proceeded to image his pancreas, but transabdominal ultrasonography, CT scanning and MRI scanning showed no abnormality. He, thereafter, underwent an endoscopic ultrasound which revealed two 5 mm × 5 mm lesions near the tail of the pancreas. A surgical opinion was sought and he underwent a distal pancreatectomy and made an uneventful recovery. Histopathology confirmed insulinoma.

INTRODUCTION TO HYPOGLYCEMIA

Hypoglycemia is defined as blood glucose less than 72 mg/dL and is commonly encountered in diabetic patients on insulin or sulfonylureas. However, hypoglycemia is seen in nondiabetic patients too due to a variety of reasons such as:
- Septic shock
- Cardiac, renal and hepatic failure
- Substance abuse (like cocaine, ethanol, etc.)
- Drugs (insulin, sulfonylureas, fluoroquinolones, salicylates, etc.)

- Adrenocortical insufficiency
- Hypopituitarism
- Tumors-like insulinoma
- Paraneoplastic syndromes
- Factitious.

Symptoms of hypoglycemia may be categorized as adrenergic or neuroglycopenic. Sympathoadrenal activation symptoms include sweating, shakiness, tachycardia, anxiety and a sensation of hunger. Neuroglycopenic symptoms include weakness, tiredness, or dizziness, inappropriate behavior (sometimes mistaken for inebriation), difficulty with concentration, confusion, blurred vision and, in extreme cases, coma and death.

Since the consequences of hypoglycemia can be devastating and an antidote is readily available, diagnosis and treatment must be rapid in any patient with suspected hypoglycemia, regardless of the cause. Patients with no previous history of hypoglycemia require a complete workup to find a potentially treatable disease.

WORKUP FOR HYPOGLYCEMIA

A careful history is essential in the workup for hypoglycemia. Symptoms such as weight loss, nausea, vomiting, sleepiness and headaches must be actively searched for. Symptoms for an infective source must be sought as should be a detailed history of hepatic renal and cardiac disease as well as diabetes. Drug history and history of substance abuse must be elicited. A family history of diabetes and other endocrinopathies as well as metabolic disorders must be documented. Clinical examination focusing on signs of sepsis, malignancy, endocrine and autoimmune diseases (like vitiligo) is essential.

Investigations should primarily look for signs of sepsis (CBC, CRP, cultures and urinalysis) and signs of malignancy (chest X-ray, abdominal imaging). Renal function and liver function tests are performed to exclude hepatic and renal impairment while an ECG and echocardiogram are performed to exclude heart failure. Serum electrolytes and thyroid function are performed to look for adrenal, pituitary and thyroid disorders. Serum cortisol measured during a hypoglycemic episode is necessary to diagnose adrenocortical failure or pituitary dysfunction. A post-synacthen stimulated cortisol level should be measured if adrenocortical insufficiency is suspected. This test is relatively difficult to perform due to poor availability of Synacthen.

Tumors of the pancreas, insulinoma, are not common but must be excluded. If hypoglycemia is not spontaneous then Whipple's triad (low blood glucose, symptoms of hypoglycemia with low blood glucose, and alleviation of symptoms with treatment of low blood glucose) must be demonstrated after a prolonged fast and when blood glucose drops below 45 mg/dL, serum insulin and C-peptide should be measured. Proinsulin levels should be measured if possible. Where these tests are available, a urinary screen for drugs, substances and sulfonylureas may be performed. Interpretations of these results are tabulated in Table 1.

IMAGING FOR INSULINOMA

Imaging plays a pivotal role in the diagnosis of insulinoma. However which mode of imaging provides the highest diagnostic yield is debatable.

Transabdominal ultrasonography is cheap and easily available and according to some studies have a 67% success rate of localizing the tumors. Some authors however disagree and put the figure far lower.

TABLE 1: Levels of insulin, C-peptide, proinsulin and urinary sulfonylurea in various cases of hypoglycemia.

Diagnosis	Symptoms or signs	Glucose (mg/dL)	Insulin (µu/mL)	C-peptide (nmol/L)	Proinsulin (pmol/L)	Sulfonylurea (urine)
Normal	No	>40	<6	<0.2	<5	No
Insulinoma	Yes	≤45	≥6	≥0.2	≥5	No
Factitious (insulin)	Yes	≤45	≥6	<0.2	<5	No
Factitious (sulfonylurea)	Yes	≤45	≥6	≥0.2	≥5	Yes
Insulin-like growth factor mediated	Yes	≤45	≤6	<0.2	<5	No
Noninsulin mediated	Yes	≤45	<6	<0.2	<5	No
Nonhypoglycemic disorder	Yes	>40	<6	<0.2	<5	No

Intraoperative ultrasonography is now touted as the imaging study of choice for its anatomical precision. It has an advantage over preoperative transabdominal ultrasound, but many surgeons prefer to know the location of the tumor before surgery. There is a long learning curve. Endoscopic ultrasound was reported in one study to have up to a 93% sensitivity and is certainly attractive with its relative noninvasiveness and superior anatomical precision compared with transabdominal ultrasound. Availability and operator dependence remain drawbacks.

The CT scanning is cheap and widely available but the diagnostic yield of CT scans is variable depending on the size of the tumor. MRI scanning and angiography have shown 87% sensitivity and 100% specificity in the diagnosis of insulinoma in one study but these findings have not been replicated.

Newer methods like octreotide scanning, arteriography, transhepatic portal venous sampling, and selective arterial calcium stimulation with venous sampling are invasive, expensive and not widely available and as of now do not seem to have enough advantages over the old methods.

In most pancreatic neuroendocrine tumors, the usefulness of positron emission tomography (PET) with fluorine-labeled fluorodeoxyglucose [(^{18}F)FDG] for lesion detection is limited because of the low glucose turnover of these tumors. Based on the capacity of pancreatic beta cells to take up and decarboxylate amine precursors, several investigators have studied patients with insulinomas using amino acid precursors, such as [^{18}F]dihydroxyphenylalanine (DOPA) and [^{11}C]hydroxytryptophan (5-HTP), in an attempt to increase the sensitivity of PET scanning. Another characteristic of neuroendocrine tumors is the expression of somatostatin receptors, and thus encouraging studies with somatostatin receptor imaging with [^{18}Ga]-labeled somatostatin analogs have emerged as a new interesting imaging tool for the diagnosis of pancreatic neuroendocrine tumors. However, this remains largely a research tool and its application in a clinical setting seems at a distance, as of now.

DISCUSSION

This patient highlights a not so common scenario—hypoglycemia in a nondiabetic patient. Hypoglycemia in patient who are not taking insulin or other drugs needs careful workup and treatment and the following review details these aspects of care.

> **Take Home Messages**
> - *Hypoglycemia in nondiabetics is uncommon and needs careful workup preferable as an inpatient and under an endocrinologist*
> - *Demonstration of the Whipple's triad is the first step in diagnosing the cause of hypoglycemia*
> - *Measurement of hormone levels when the patient is hypoglycemic provides key information as to the cause of hypoglycemia*
> - *Treatment is focused on the cause of hypoglycemia.*

SUGGESTED READING

1. Grant C. Insulinoma. Best Pract Res Clin Gastroenterol. 2005;19:783-9.
2. Hamdy O, Srinivasan VAR, Snow KJ, et al. (2019). Hypoglycemia. [online] Available from http://emedicine.medscape.com/article/122122-overview [Last accessed June, 2019].
3. Kauhannen S, Sepannen M, Minn H, et al. Clinical PET Imaging of Insulinoma and Beta-Cell Hyperplasia. Curr Pharma Design. 2010;16:1550-60.
4. Marney A, Jagasia S. Case Study: Diagnostic Dilemma in a Patient with Insulinoma. Clin Diab. 2007;25:152-4.
5. Okabayashi T, Shima Y, Sumioshi T, et al. Diagnosis and Management of Insulinoma. World J Gastroenterol. 2013;19(6):829-37.
6. Service JF. Hypoglycemic disorders. N Engl J Med. 1995;333:1144-52.

SECTION 10

Parathyroid

CASE 1: Brown Tumor of the Lower Jaw as the First Manifestation of Primary Hyperparathyroidism: A Case Report

Subir Ray

CASE HISTORY

A 48-year-old male patient presented to the maxillofacial department of our hospital with the complaints of increasing swelling in the left side of lower jaw with pain and loosening of the adjacent teeth of 2–3 months duration (Fig. 1). His past medical history included well-controlled type 2 diabetes mellitus (T2DM), systemic hypertension, dyslipidemia and subclinical hypothyroidism. There was no history of renal calculi. An X-ray of mandible showed a radiolucent lesion of the mandible extending from left premolar region with irregular margins and evidence of root resorption.

Blood tests showed elevated adjusted serum calcium level 13.4 mg/dL (normal range, 8.2–10.2), phosphorous 1.8 mg/dL (normal range 2.5–4 ng/dL), alkaline phosphatase 236 IU/L (normal range up to 100) and intact parathormone 460 pg/mL (normal range, 15–65). Sestamibi scan of the parathyroid glands revealed parathyroid adenoma in the lower pole of the right lobe of the thyroid gland. Right inferior parathyroidectomy was performed and immediate postoperative iPTH level was 90 pg/mL. Patient was discharged with calcium and alpha-calcidol and followed up after 4 weeks. His repeat blood biochemistry showed adjusted calcium 9.1 mg/dL phosphorous 2.8 mg/dL, and iPTH 23 pg/mL. Repeat X-rays done showed steady regression of the lytic lesion which almost disappeared after 6 months. In view of his normal blood biochemistry, calcium and alpha-calcidol were stopped after 6 months.

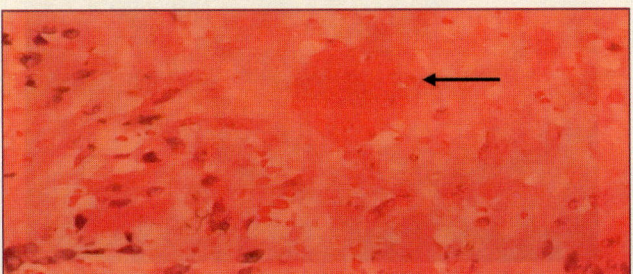

FIG. 1: Hematoxylin and eosin (H&E) stain of the gingival mass showing giant cell granuloma (blue arrow) on light microscopy.

INTRODUCTION

Primary HPT is a condition where there is overproduction of parathyroid hormone (PTH) by one or more hyperfunctioning parathyroid glands resulting in hypercalcemia. Majority (80–90%) are caused by a single parathyroid adenoma and the rest are caused by parathyroid hyperplasia. Virtually 99% of the adenomas are benign. Commonly the patients are asymptomatic initially and diagnosis is incidental. Occasionally patients may present with including renal stones, osteoporosis, neuropsychiatric symptoms and, rarely, pancreatitis. Brown tumors are focal giant cell lesion resulting from areas of abnormal bone resorption, which is replaced by fibrovascular tissue and giant cells with plenty of hemosiderin deposits. This is not a very common presenting feature of primary HPT. Different imaging techniques, e.g. ultrasonography of abdomen and neck, CT scan and technetium-99m (Tc-99m) may be useful in diagnosis and localizing the offending adenoma and the bony lesion.

DISCUSSION

Brown tumors are normally a later presentation of primary HPT. They occur due to imbalance of osteoclastic and osteoblastic activity resulting in formation of bony cavities which get filled up by fibrous tissues. Mandibular involvement is uncommon but not rare. But it is a rare first clinical manifestation of primary HPT before the onset of general manifestations. Clinically, brown tumors of the mandible present as painful, hard swelling and radiographically, as well-defined monolocular or multilocular osteolytic lesions with root resorption.

Diagnosis of primary PTH is confirmed by establishing hypercalcemia and elevated parathyroid hormone levels. Tc-99m sestamibi scanning is very helpful for preoperative localization.

Treatment of symptomatic primary HPT is surgical removal of the parathyroid adenoma. Spontaneous regression of smaller osteolytic lesions is common after parathyroidectomy as happened in this case but disfiguring large lesions may need excision. Surgical excision of the jaw lesion, if needed, is usually done after parathyroid surgery.

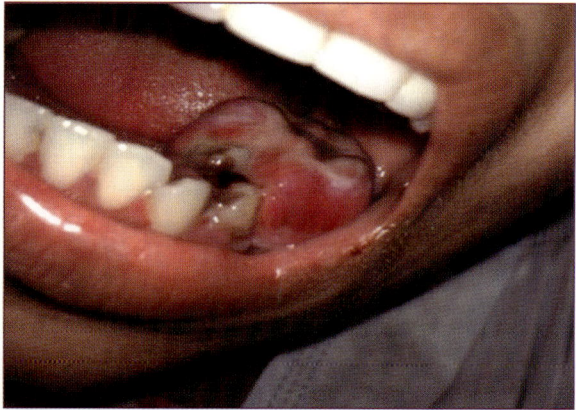

FIG. 2: Left mandibular mass.

Take Home Message

- Brown tumor of hyperparathyroidism should be considered in cases of radiolucent jaw tumors or tumors showing giant cells on histopathology as many of them may not require surgery and completely resolve after parathyroidectomy (Fig. 2).

SUGGESTED READING

1. Fraser WD. Hyperparathyroidism. Lancet. 2009;374:145-58.
2. Rosenberg EH, Guralnick WC. Hyperparathyroidism: a review of 220 proved cases, with special emphasis on findings in the jaws. Oral Surg. 1962;15:83.
3. Shetty AD, Namitha J, James L. Brown Tumor of Mandible in Association with Primary Hyperparathyroidism: A Case Report. J Int Oral Health. 2015;7(2):50-2.
4. Suarez-Cunqueiro MM, Schoen R, Kersten A, et al. Brown tumor of the mandible as first manifestation of atypical parathyroid adenoma. J Oral Maxillofac Surg. 2004;62:1024-8.

CASE 2 | An Interesting Case of Acute Confusional State

Sujoy Majumdar

CASE HISTORY

An 80-year-old male, a known patient of type 2 diabetes mellitus (T2DM), hypothyroidism and hypertension presented to the hospital emergency room (ER) with worsening of level of consciousness over last 7 days. Other medical problems included untreated prostatic hyperplasia and a left-sided inguinal hernia. About 3 years ago, he had sustained a fall at home and developed bilateral subdural hematoma which was evacuated by Burr Hole surgery. Since then he had a fluctuating level of consciousness and had been mostly bed bound. A provisional diagnosis of vascular dementia and parkinsonism was made by the local physician. Over the last 48 hours he had been doubly incontinent and had been taking very little food or drinks. List of medicines included injection human mixtard (PreMix biphasic insulin), metformin, levothyroxine, amlodipine, telmisartan, atorvastatin, levodopa and carbidopa.

On examination, he was alert but disoriented to time, place and person. There was clinically no pallor, cyanosis or jaundice but looked clinically dehydrated. Temperature was 99°F, HR: 97 beats/min in sinus rhythm and BP: 140/90 mm Hg. No neurological abnormality was noted except some generalized weakness (power grade 4/5 in all four limbs). Examination of cardiovascular and respiratory system was noncontributory. Nonspecific abdominal tenderness could be elicited. Rest of the examination was unremarkable.

Investigations: The relevant initial investigations are shown in Table 1.

TABLE 1: Investigations done post admission.

Hemoglobin	14.5 g/dL	Serum creatinine	2.1 mg/dL (eGFR = 31 mL/min/1.73 m^2)
PCV	42.4%	Calcium	16.2 mg/dL
MCV	77.9 fL	Albumin	4.1 g/dL
MCH	26.7 pg	Corrected calcium	16.1 g/dL
TLC	11,920/mm^3	Phosphate	2.1 g/dL
Neutrophil	83%	SGPT	28 U/L
Lymphocytes	14%	SGOT	32 U/L
Monocytes	3%	Bilirubin	0.9 mg/dL
Eosinophils	0%	PSA	2.35 ng/mL
ESR	10	Free T4	1.7 ng/dL
CRP	15	TSH	4.8 µIU/mL
HbA1c	7.2%	Urine RE/ME	Absent glucose and ketone; Pus cells: 20–22/hpf
FPG	120 mg/dL		
PPPG	127 mg/dL	Urine C/S	Growth of *Escherichia coli* (10^5 cfu/mL)
Serum sodium/potassium	129/3.8 mmol/L	Chest X-ray and 12-lead ECG	Unremarkable
USG abdomen	Bilateral renal parenchymal disease with multiple renal cysts and left-sided nephrolithiasis. Marked prostatic enlargement (82.4 g) with post void residual urine volume of 75 mL		
CT scan of brain	Ill-defined hypodensities in bilateral frontal and periventricular and subcortical white matter consistent with mild diffuse cerebral atrophy with ischemic changes		

(HbA1c: glycosylated hemoglobin; PCV: packed cell volume; MCV: mean corpuscular volume; MCH: mean cell hemoglobin; TLC: total leukocyte count; ESR: erythrocyte sedimentation rate; CRP: C-reactive protein; FPG: fasting plasma glucose; PPPG: postprandial plasma glucose; SGPT: serum glutamic pyruvic transaminase; SGOT: serum glutamic oxaloacetic transaminase; PSA: prostate-specific antigen; TSH: thyroid-stimulating hormone ECG: electrocardiogram; USG: ultrasonography; RE: routine examination; ME: microbial examination)

Question 1: What is the diagnosis?

Answer: The obvious major abnormality is hypercalcemia with chronic kidney disease. Urosepsis along with obstructive uropathy in the presence of diabetes and hypertension could be the possible causes for the deteriorating renal function.

Causes of hypercalcemia are shown in Box 1.

Box 1: Causes of hypercalcemia.

- Malignancy: Multiple myeloma, metastases from systemic malignancy
- Endocrine: Hyperparathyroidism (the most common)

Acromegaly, hyperthyroidism, Addison's disease (rare causes)

- Renal failure with tertiary hyperparathyroidism
- Sarcoidosis and other granulomatous diseases
- Paget's disease
- Prolonged immobilization
- Excessive lithium intake
- Vitamin D intoxication
- Familial hypocalciuric hypocalcemia

Question 2: What other tests were done to confirm the diagnosis?

Answer: The other tests done to confirm the diagnosis are shown in Box 2.

Box 2: Diagnostic investigations for final diagnosis.

- X-ray skull, spine and pelvis did not show any lytic lesions
- *Serum protein electrophoresis*: Within normal limits. No "monoclonal" peak noted either in the γ or β region. There was a minimal elevation of β1 region, corresponding with infection
- *25(OH) vitamin D*: 42 ng/mL
- *Intact PTH (iPTH) (done by ECILA method)*: 562.29 pg/mL (NR: 15–65 pg/mL)
- *USG of neck*: An encapsulated solid SOL, poster-inferior to the right lobe of thyroid measuring approximately 1.22 cm × 1.16 cm, having an isoechoic center with hypoechoic peripheral rim, consistent with a right-sided parathyroid adenoma. No other abnormality was noted (Fig. 1)
- *Technetium-99m (Tc-99m) sestamibi scan of parathyroid*: It confirms the presence of a well-defined area of increased uptake with delayed washout in the above area of SOL with no features on increased uptake in any other area (Fig. 2)

Final diagnosis: Hypercalcemia due to parathyroid adenoma with nephrolithiasis with acute on chronic renal failure in a case of diabetes with hypertension and hypothyroidism.

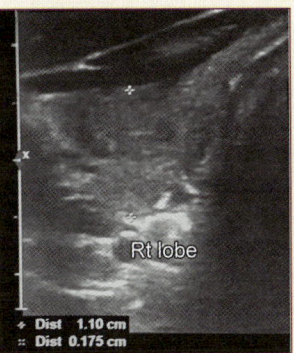

FIG. 1: USG neck demonstrating the parathyroid adenoma.

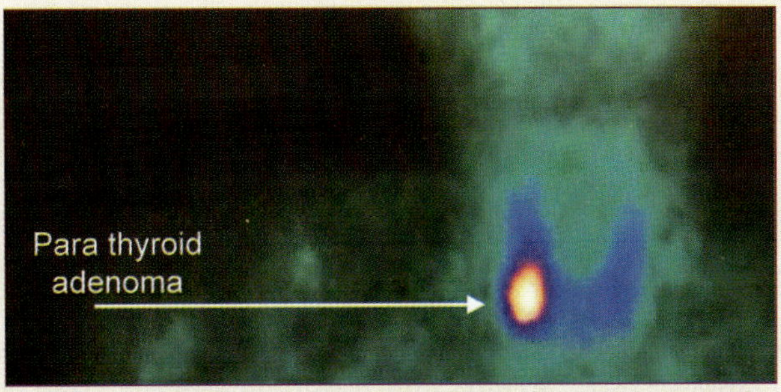

FIG. 2: Technetium-99m (Tc-99m) sestamibi scan showing the presence of parathyroid adenoma.

INTRODUCTION

Acute confusional state often presents as a diagnostic dilemma for the practicing physician symptomatic hyperparathyroidism constitutes an important but often underdiagnosed cause in the differential diagnosis (Box 3).

MANAGEMENT

Patient was treated with intravenous (IV) normal saline, followed by IV frusemide for hypercalcemia. Bisphosphonates could not be used as the renal function kept on worsening (serum creatinine went up to 3.4 mg/dL). Glycemic control was obtained with IV insulin infusion pump. Urinary tract infection was controlled with IV antibiotics. BP was stabilized with antihypertensives. Hypothyroidism was managed with levothyroxine replacement. Despite the optimal treatment, patient's corrected calcium did not drop lower than 12.5 mg/dL. Serum creatinine reduced to 1.6 mg/dL. Patient subsequently underwent

> **Box 3: Common causes of acute confusional state.**
> - *Infections*: Sepsis resulting from pneumonia, urinary tract infection, disseminated skin infections, meningoencephalitis, cerebral malaria and dengue
> - *Drugs*: Alcohol and alcohol withdrawal, narcotic drugs, ketamine, benzodiazepines, pesticides, anticholinergics
> - *Metabolic*:
>   - Diabetic ketoacidosis, hyperosmolar coma, hypoglycemia, hyponatremia, hypernatremia, hypercalcemia, hypocalcemia, hypomagnesemia
>   - Type 2 respiratory failure with hypercarbia
>   - Hepatic encephalopathy
>   - Chronic kidney disease with uremic encephalopathy
>   - Gross dehydration from diarrhea and vomiting
> - *Endocrine*: Hyperthyroidism, hypothyroidism, hyperparathyroidism, addison's disease, acromegaly
> - *Neurological*: Cerebrovascular accident (hemorrhage/large infarct), intracranial neoplastic lesion with hemorrhage, hypertensive encephalopathy, CNS vasculitis

resection of the right parathyroid adenoma under general anesthesia. His serum calcium levels started coming down within the next 24 hours and had to be corrected with IV calcium gluconate and calcitriol. Patient's level of consciousness improved significantly. He was discharged after 7 days with a serum calcium (corrected): 9.1 mg/dL, phosphate: 3.4 mg/dL and serum creatinine: 1.3 mg/dL.

DISCUSSION

Hyperparathyroidism is caused by a single gland adenoma in 80% of cases. Lesser common causes include four gland hyperplasia (10–15%) and parathyroid carcinoma (<5% cases). Parathyroid adenomas occur more commonly in lower pole (as was seen in the case). Ectopic adenomas, though extremely rare, can occur in thymus. Hyperparathyroidism is a disease of the elderly, the incidence being 2% in those above 55 years of age. Classical features of primary hyperparathyroidism are kidney disease (nephrolithiasis, rarely nephrocalcinosis and renal impairment) and bone disease (osteoporosis particularly involving cortical bone, osteitis fibrosa cystic and brown tumors), vitamin D deficiency, due to increased clearance of 25(OH) vitamin D under the influence of high PTH levels, can result in proximal myopathy. However, classical features with the exception of nephrolithiasis are now uncommon.

Corrected calcium (for albumin) is assessed by the following equation:

Corrected calcium (in mg/dL) = Measured total calcium (in mg/dL) + 0.8 × (4 − patient's serum albumin in g/L)

The primary modality of medical management is:
- Correction of hypercalcemia by IV normal saline and loop diuretics. Typical fluid regime is 1 L normal saline every 6–8 hourly. Fluid resuscitation alone will reduce serum calcium by up to 2 mg/dL
- Use and dosage of loop diuretics have to be carefully planned in order to avoid unnecessary volume depletion
- IV bisphosphonates are indicated for long-term control of hypercalcemia if eGFR >60 mL/min/1.73 m² and are to be avoided below eGFR 30 mL/min. Zolendronic acid is preferred to pamidronate. It is particularly helpful in those with low bone mass

- Cinacalcet is indicated as a part of medical management in patients unfit for surgery, when corrected serum calcium is >12 mg/dL.

Definitive treatment for symptomatic disease (if patient is fit) is parathyroidectomy. For asymptomatic disease, surgery is indicated if:
- Age <50 years
- Serum calcium (corrected) >11.6 mg/dL
- History of pathological fracture
- Presence of nephrocalcinosis/nephrolithiasis
- DEXA scan T-score <2.5
- Progressive decline of eGFR <60 mL/min.

Success of surgery depends on the surgeon's skill, experience and correct preoperative decision making.

Postoperative "hungry bone syndrome" manifested by symptomatic and biochemical hypocalcemia occurs in 75% patients, particularly in those with overt bone disease. Risk of "hungry bone syndrome" is proportional to the initial serum calcium. The maximal fall of serum calcium occurs between 12 hours to 3 days. Initial treatment is IV calcium infusion and calcitriol. Long-term oral calcium supplementation is necessary.

Take Home Messages

- *A persistent confusional state in a patient following successful evacuation of a subdural hematoma should not be dismissed as simply due to a multi-infarct state*
- *Proper metabolic work-up for causes outlined in Box 1 is necessary*
- *Primary hyperparathyroidism constitutes a relatively rare but potentially curable case of confusional case.*

SUGGESTED READING

1. Bilezikian JP, Khan AA, Potts JT, et al. Guidelines for management of asymptomatic primary hyperparathyroidism: summary statement—3rd International Workshop. J Clin Endocrinol Metab. 2009;94:335-9.
2. Cooper MS. Disorders of calcium metabolism and parathyroid disease. Best Pract Res Clin Endocrinol Metab. 2011;25:975-83.
3. Endre DB. Investigations of hypercalcemia. Clin Biochem. 2012;45:954-63.
4. Marcocci C, Cetani F. Primary hyperparathyroidism. N Engl J Med. 2005;352:373-79.
5. Yu N, Leese GP, Donnan PT. What predicts adverse outcome in untreated primary hyperparathyroidism? The Parathyroid Epidemiology and Audit Research Study (PEARS). Clin Endocrinol. 2013;79:27-34.

SECTION 11

Pituitary

CASE 1: Uncontrolled Hyperglycemia–Think beyond Glycemia

Animesh Maiti, Anirban Sinha, Asish Kumar Basu, Partha Sarathi Choudhury, Saurav Shishir, Chhavi Agrawal

CASE HISTORY

A 56-year-old male hypertensive with diabetes mellitus for last 1 year presented with poorly controlled hyperglycemia even on multiple OHAs. In retrospect, he had associated with complaints of polyarthralgia (involving elbow joints, wrist joints and knee joints), dull aching headache and snoring during sleep for last 5 months. He also had complaints of excessive sweating and tingling sensation in bilateral lower limbs along with reduced libido and erectile dysfunction for last 1 year. His father was a known diabetic.

The clinical examinations are summarized in Table 1. Patient had prognathism, large fleshy nose, prominent nasolabial folds and thick lower lips, macroglossia, seborrhea and

TABLE 1: Clinical examination.

Parameters	Value
Pulse rate	84 beats/min
Blood pressure	164/80 mm Hg
Weight	66.5 kg
Height	167.2 cm
Body mass index	23.78 kg/m^2
Waist circumference	83 cm
Hip circumference	90 cm
Acanthosis	Grade 2
Hormonal evaluation	
Thyroid-stimulating hormone/free thyroxin	1.04 mIU/L/1.17 ng/dL
Prolactin	739.2 ng/mL
Insulin-like growth factor 1 (after achieving normoglycemia)	412 ng/mL (36–188 ng/mL)
Cortisol	8.77 µg/dL
Growth hormone suppression test with 75 g oral glucose	7 ng/mL (not suppressed)

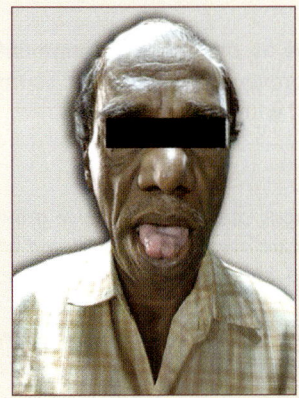

FIG. 1: Coarse facial features with macroglossia.

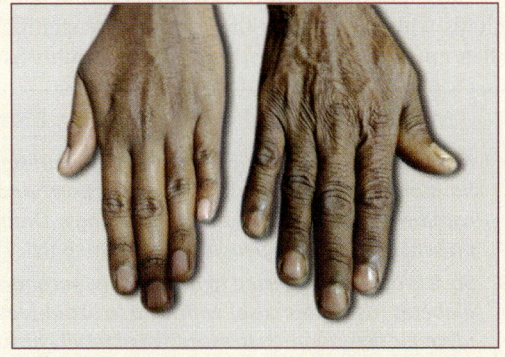

FIG. 2: Spade like hand (right side).

multiple skin tags (Fig. 1). He had spade like hands and feet along with increased heel pad thickness (Fig. 2). Testes: 25 mL and soft in consistency bilaterally. Confrontation perimetry test revealed right temporal field defect.

MRI pituitary showed pituitary macroadenoma (KNOSP Grade 3, HARDY IV E) (Fig. 3).

Automated perimetry detected a right temporal field defect.

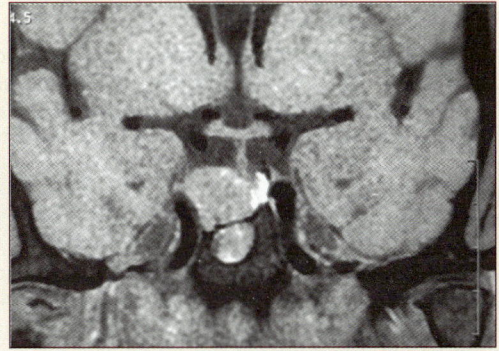

FIG. 3: MRI pituitary showing pituitary macroadenoma.

DIAGNOSIS

A case of probable type 2 diabetes mellitus (T2DM) with uncontrolled hyperglycemia secondary to active acromegaly due to pituitary macroadenoma.

DISCUSSION

Acromegaly comprises a collection of symptoms and signs caused by excessive growth hormone (GH) secretion that leads to bony and soft tissue overgrowth associated with cardiovascular and metabolic pathology. Diabetes and impaired glucose tolerance is present in 15–38% of people with acromegaly.

So, it is always suggested to rule out any secondary cause like acromegaly in patients with diabetes (as in this case) with coarse facial features and acral enlargement with recent glycemic deterioration irrespective of family history.

Moreover, it is also suggested to measure IGF-1 in patients without having the typical manifestations of acromegaly, but who have several of these associated conditions, e.g.

sleep apnea syndrome, T2DM, debilitating arthritis, carpal tunnel syndrome, hyperhidrosis and hypertension.

Trans-sphenoidal pituitary surgery is recommended as the primary treatment in patients with acromegaly that can lead to significant improvement in glycemic status as well as amelioration in morbidity and mortality associated with acromegaly.

Take Home Messages

- Acromegaly comprises a collection of symptoms and signs caused by excessive growth hormone (GH) secretion that leads to bony and soft tissue overgrowth associated with cardiovascular and metabolic pathology. Diabetes and impaired glucose tolerance is present in 15–38% of people with acromegaly
- So, it is always suggested to rule out any secondary cause like acromegaly in patients with diabetes (as in this case) with coarse facial features and acral enlargement with recent glycemic deterioration irrespective of family history
- Moreover, it is also suggested to measure IGF-1 in patients without having the typical manifestations of acromegaly, but who have several of these associated conditions, e.g. sleep apnea syndrome, T2DM, debilitating arthritis, carpal tunnel syndrome, hyperhidrosis and hypertension
- Transsphenoidal pituitary surgery is recommended as the primary treatment in patients with acromegaly that can lead to significant improvement in glycemic status as well as amelioration in morbidity and mortality associated with acromegaly.

SUGGESTED READING

1. DeGroot's Text book of Endocrinology. 7th edition.
2. Harrison's Text book of Internal Medicine.19th edition. November 2014.
3. Melmed S, Polonsky KS, Larsen PR, Kronenberg HM. William's Text book of Endocrinology. 13th edition. January 2016.

CASE 2 | Hot Flashes in Men: Rare Presentation of a Rare Disorder

Biswajit Ghoshdastidar

CASE HISTORY

A 57-year-old gentleman, a British council clerk, presented with history of intermittent episodes of heat intolerance and sweating, progressive weakness, anorexia, occasional vomiting and nonproductive cough with wheeze. He was well until about a month ago and was on no long-term medication and a recent health check-up (2 months back) revealed no significant abnormality except low normal thyroid-stimulating hormone (TSH). On the day of hospitalization, he felt exceptionally unwell, profusely sweating and BP was 100/60 mm Hg. He was clinically dehydrated and systemic examination was otherwise normal except bilateral rhonchi.

Investigation revealed the following.	
Thyroid-stimulating hormone	0.12 mIU/mL
Free thyroxine	0.09 ng/mL
Free triiodothyronine	2.41 pmol/L
Total testosterone	100 ng/dL (Low)
Luteinizing hormone	1.48 IU/L (1.5–9.3) (Low)
Follicle-stimulating hormone	4.23 IU/mL (1.4–18.1)
Prolactin	8.13 ng/mL (2.1–17.7)
Serum sodium	129 mEq/L
Serum potassium	4.6 mEq/L
Mantoux	Positive
Cortisol AM	0.25 µg/dL (Low)
Cortisol PM	0.15 µg/dL (Low)
8 AM adrenocorticotropic hormone	13.1 pg/mL (Low normal)
Serum creatinine	1.31 mg/dL
Chest X-ray	Normal
Visual field test (Perimetry)	Normal

WORKING DIAGNOSIS: AUTOIMMUNE HYPOPHYSITIS

Dramatic clinical improvement (in term of sense of well being) took place with corticosteroid (IV followed by oral) supplementation and subsequently L-thyroxine replacement. Hot flashes (his most distressing symptoms) improved in severity and frequency and almost disappeared after 1 month.

DISCUSSION

Hot Flashes in Men

About 70% of women experience hot flashes around the time of menopause; due to dip in the estrogen level. In men, after the age of 40 years, testosterone level drops by around 1% every year and since the decline is gradual and even at the advanced age, the level is still within normal level and hence men do not experience hot flashes. However, in situation, where testosterone level drops precipitously, men may experience hot flashes along with other symptom of androgen deficiency. One common situation is drug-induced testosterone deficiency as a part of treatment of carcinoma prostrate drugs such as, leuprolide or goserelin (which competitively block of the release of gonadotropin releasing hormone) or drug like bicalutamide that blocks the effect of testosterone on tissues.

Hot flashes are an unusual presentation in autoimmune hypophysitis and more common presentation is headache. In this particular case, pituitary was only moderately enlarged and hence perhaps did not produce headache or visual disturbances, as suggested by normal visual perimeter. On the contrary, pituitary hypofunction was considerable, notably very low cortisol, LH, testosterone and Free T4 level. TB and sarcoid, as etiology, was unlikely. mantoux positive with 15 mm induration was obviously inconclusive and normal SACE and a normal chest X-ray in the absence of other clinical features of sarcoidosis ruled out the necessity of any further investigation at this stage of illness. Etiological definitive diagnosis is only possible, when surgical treatment (decompression) is required. In this case, the symptoms rapidly improved after initiation of corticosteroid treatment, surgical intervention was not required and a working diagnosis of autoimmune hypophysitis was made.

Clinical Suspicion of Hypophysitis

Symptom and Sign
Early: Headache, visual impairment, nausea, vomiting, loss of appetite, fatigue, weakness, asthenia, fever, lethargy, hypotension, hypoglycemia, hyponatremia and eosinophilia.
Late: Amenorrhea, impotence and coma.

Consider Adrenal Insufficiency (Fig. 1)

Diagnostic tests: Brain MRI, blood pressure, ECG, glycemia, plasma osmolality, electrolytes, blood cell count, ACTH, TSH, IGF-L, FSH, LH, ADH, cortisol, Free T4, prolactin, testosterone/estradiol and visual field.

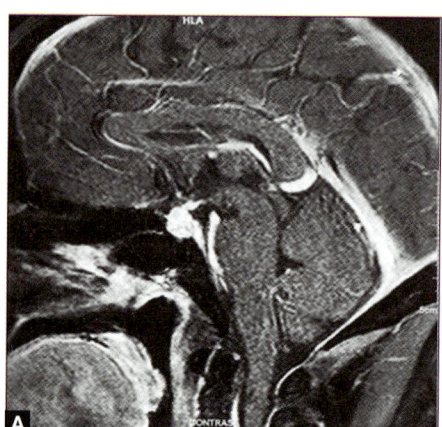 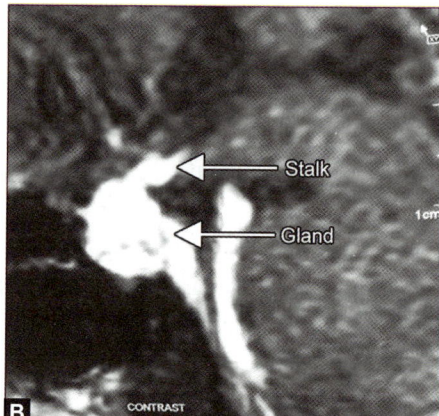

FIG. 1: MRI (A) Brain; (B) Bulky pituitary gland and stalk (no mass lesion).

Endocrinology Consultation

Treatment: Steroid replacement therapy and debulking with surgery for expanding sellar masses unresponsive to medical treatment.

> **Take Home Message**
>
> - This relatively rare disorder can occur in both women and men and is not necessarily only provoked by pregnancy. CTLA-4 blockade (Monoclonal antibody treatment, quite frequently used drug in many cancers, nowadays) is notoriously associated with this condition and hence etiology and clinical presentation of this unique disease are likely to be expanding and physicians in the primary care should lower the threshold of suspicion in a case presenting with headache and features of hypopituitarism in clinical practice; keeping in mind that rare presentation, as in this case, can be quite puzzling at times.

SUGGESTED READING

1. Harrison's Principles of Internal Medicine, 19th edition. p. 2257.
2. Luliano SL, Laws ER. The Diagnosis and Management of Lymphocytic Hypophysitis. Expert Rev Endocrinol Metab. 2011;6(6):777-83.

CASE 3: Snake and the Pituitary

Kalyan Kumar Gangopadhyay

CASE HISTORY

A 65-year-old farmer was admitted with a history of snake bite over his right index finger while doing agricultural work. The species of snake, however, was not identified. He complained of swelling and severe burning sensation at the site of the bite. He was immediately taken to a local hospital, where he was given 10 vials of anti-snake venom (ASV) IV, and was transferred to our tertiary care hospital.

After admission, he received further doses of ASV. Because of clotting abnormalities he received fresh frozen plasma. Table 1 below shows the laboratory tests done since admission.

Because of deteriorating renal function he received intermittent hemodialysis. This is common in viper snake bite which causes intravascular hemolysis. As it can be seen in

TABLE 1: Some of the relevant laboratory tests done since admission.

Date	Serum sodium	Serum potassium	Serum creatinine	Others
Day 1	137	3.3	1.6	Clotting time >10 min
Day 2		3.4	3.42	
Day 4		3	5.32	
Day 5		3.1	6.26	
Day 6				Drop in hemoglobin from 13 on admission to 8.9
Day 8	134	3.6	6.96	
Day 10	132	3.3	9.5	
Day 11		3.8	10.77	
Day 12	125	3.7	8.4	
Day 13	122	4.8	8.87	
Day 15	122	4.8		TSH 0.118 µIU/mL
Day 16				T3 = 0.453 ng/dL (0.8–2.0)
				T4 = 3.29 µg/dL (4.6–12)
				Cortisol 4.8 µg/dL
Day 17				LH 0.1 mIU/mL. MRI pituitary Hydrocortisone started
Day 19	134			Thyroid replacement started

(LH: luteinizing hormone; TSH: thyroid-stimulating hormone; MRI: magnetic resonance imaging)

Table 1, he developed an unexplained drop in sodium 12 days after admission. Endocrine profile suggested hypopituitarism and was promptly started on hydrocortisone which was subsequently maintained on 20 mg at 7 AM and 10 mg at 4 PM. Thyroid replacement was also started at 25 µg thyroxine, which was gradually increased to 50 after 1 week. MRI pituitary was done which showed degeneration of anterior pituitary and loss of normal signal pattern on T1-weighted images.

The patient came for follow-up after 2 months and a short Synacthen test was done which revealed a 30 minutes cortisol of 8 µg/dL and a TSH of 0.12 µIU/mL suggesting sustained pituitary failure. He was otherwise well and serum sodium was 138.

DISCUSSION

Prevalence

Snake bite has been recognized by the WHO as a neglected tropical disease in 2009. Snake bite claims more than 45,000 deaths annually, which is more than many of the common tropical diseases. Snake bites may lead to renal failure and associated problems of intravascular hemolysis, disseminated intravascular coagulation (DIC) may occur. Majority of the published literature highlights either mortality or renal failure.

Pituitary damage is an important but less well-known complication following snake bite. Observational studies of snake bite survivors revealed that up to 10% of patients develop pituitary damage following snake bite.

Pathogenesis

Pituitary damage from snake bite could be acute or chronic. At this point it is unclear whether delayed presentation is a result of late diagnosis of acute pituitary failure or whether there is progressive destruction over months or years. Acute pituitary damage could be as a result of direct effect of the toxin, increased capillary permeability, DIC related microthrombosis leading to ischemic necrosis. Subsequently chronic antigen leakage may promote ongoing pituitary destruction through antibody production, eventually leading to pituitary hormone failure at a much later date.

Clinical Features

The pituitary damage from snake bite could be acute but persistent, however as mentioned above it could manifest at a later date. In fact the lag period between onset of pituitary damage and envenomation is wide, ranging from a few hours to a few years, with patients presenting as late as 15 years after snake bite. Of all the cases published in literature around 50% present as acute and 50% present at a later date.

The hormonal profiles predominantly affected in the acute phase were growth hormone, corticotropin, gonadotropin, thyroid hormone and prolactin, in that order. Posterior pituitary damage following snake bite is rare. These deficiencies generally persist on follow-up. Although many studies point toward acute kidney disease as a predictor of hypopituitarism, most of those studies only included patients who developed renal failure. However other studies could not find such correlation. Hence, although there are no predictors of occurrence of hypopituitarism, particular attention with regard to pituitary assessment needs to be given in patients who develop renal failure.

TABLE 2: Hormonal deficiencies and MRI findings in snake bite survivors presenting with chronic pituitary dysfunction.

Clinical features	Proportion of patients
Renal failure	70%
Hypogonadism	90–100%
Hypothyroidism	90–95%
Growth hormone deficiency	70–80%
Adrenal insufficiency	70–80%
Diabetes insipidus	5%
MRI normal	40%
MRI empty sella	35%
MRI partially empty sella	25%

In the acute phase, persistent hypotension and hyponatremia should alert the physician toward the development of pituitary failure. However, in the chronic phase, the clinical manifestations may be nonspecific as it would depend on the extent of hormone deficiency. Men presenting with delayed pituitary failure usually present with fatigue, reduced libido and weight loss and women present with fatigue, loss of appetite and secondary amenorrhea. Table 2 elaborates the hormonal deficiencies and radiological findings in patients with delayed pituitary dysfunction.

Radiological findings in chronic pituitary failure may be misleading as up to 40% may have normal pituitary on MRI examination. The rest may have either an empty sella or a partially empty sella. There is no correlation between the presence of empty sella and the severity of hormone deficiency.

Hence, the practising physician should be alert to the possibility of pituitary failure, an important but easily overlooked complication of snake bite, both in the acute phase and later on. The presence of unexplained hypotension and hyponatremia in the acute phase and a later presentation of lack of energy, loss of libido, weight loss and secondary amenorrhea should alert the physician to pituitary failure in a patient with a history of snake bite

---

Take Home Messages

- *Pituitary dysfunction may occur in up to 10% of patients with snake bite*
- *Hypopituitarism may present acutely but may also present at a much later date following snake bite*
- *Unexplained hyponatremia and hypotension following snake bite in the acute phase may point toward hypopituitary state*
- *Pituitary dysfunction in a patient with a history of snake bite should also be looked at in patients complaining of lack of energy, loss of libido, weight loss, and secondary amenorrhea.*

SUGGESTED READING

1. Golay V, Roychowdhary A, Dasgupta S, et al. Hypopituitarism in patients with vasculotoxic snake bite envenomation related acute kidney injury: a prospective study on the prevalence and outcomes of this complication. Pituitary. 2014;17(2):125-31.
2. Naik BN, Bhalla A, Sharma N, et al. Pituitary dysfunction in survivors of Russell's viper snake bite envenomation: A prospective study. Neurol India. 2018;66(5):1351-8.
3. Shivaprasad C, Aiswarya Y, Sridevi A, et al. Delayed hypopituitarism following Russell's viper envenomation: a case series and literature review. Pituitary. 2019;22(1):4-12.

CASE 4: Prolactinoma: A Rare and Treatable Cause of Male Infertility

Nilanjan Sengupta, Rahul Valsaraj

CASE HISTORY

A 35-year-old male IT professional, married for 7 months, presented to our OPD in January 2019 distressed by nonconsummation of marriage, erectile dysfunction and anejaculation. He had no history of diabetes, hypothyroidism, no habituations to ethanol or smoking and had no significant drug history. He did not give any history of headache, blurring of vision or loss of consciousness. On examination, his vitals were normal, visual testing including perimetry noncontributory, and examination of external genitalia was unremarkable in Tanner staging of P5G5A1, a testicular volume of 25 mL bilaterally and a stretched penile length of 11 cm. His systemic examination was within normal limits. The salient investigation findings are given in Table 1.

This was suggestive of hyperprolactinemia with hypogonadotropic hypogonadism. An MRI brain showed a pituitary macroadenoma (Figs. 1A and B).

TABLE 1: Investigations (January 2019).

Investigation	Report
Fasting plasma glucose	92 mg/dL
Thyroid-stimulating hormone	1.02 mIU/mL
Free thyroxine	0.93 ng/dL
8 AM cortisol	8.4 µg/dL
Plasma adrenocorticotropic hormone	38.16 pg/mL
Follicle-stimulating hormone	1.03 mIU/mL
Luteinizing hormone	0.93 mIU/mL
Total testosterone	87.5 ng/dL
Prolactin	1,238 ng/mL
Prolactin after polyethylene glycol precipitation	1,077 ng/mL

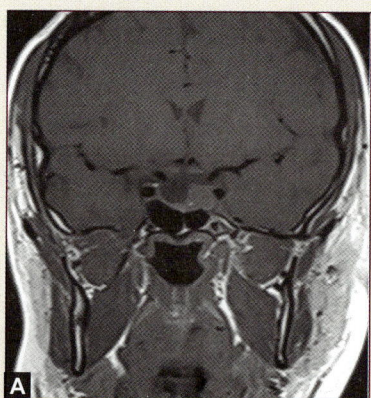
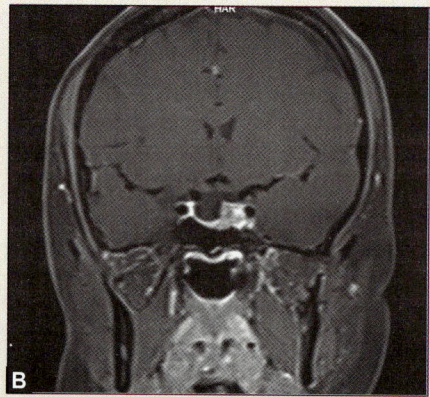

FIGS. 1A AND B: MRI brain (January 2019).

He was started on treatment with tablet cabergoline 0.5 mg twice weekly. He subsequently came for follow-up in March 2019 with marginal improvement in sexual function and the repeat investigation findings as summarized in Table 2.

TABLE 2: Investigations (March 2019).

Investigations	Report
Follicle-stimulating hormone	2.91 mIU/mL
Luteinizing hormone	1.96 mIU/mL
Prolactin	5.61 ng/mL
Total testosterone	471 ng/dL

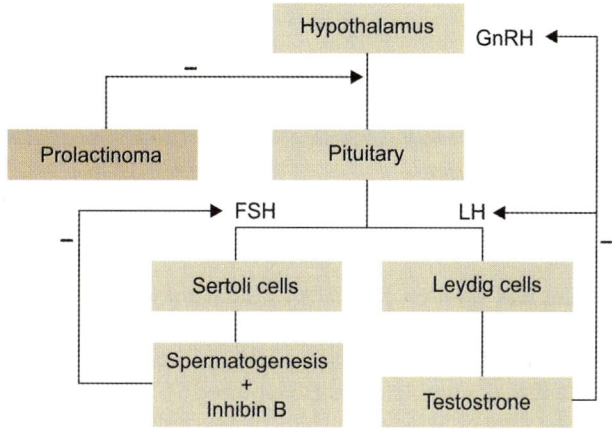

(FSH: follicle-stimulating hormone; GnRH: gonadotropin-releasing hormone; LH: luteinizing hormone)

FLOWCHART 1: Effects of prolactinoma on hypothalamic–pituitary–gonadal axis.

DISCUSSION

Hyperprolactinemia is a common cause of infertility in both sexes. Clinical presentation of the prolactinomas is earlier in females compared to males, even when they are very small (microadenoma). This earlier presentation in females is due to greater symptom of burden caused by hyperprolactinemia in them. On the other hand, males present late till prolactinoma becomes large in size (macroprolactinoma) and start causing pressure over optic chiasm and present as visual deterioration or visual field defects. They can also present with decreased libido.

Take Home Message

- The present case demonstrates that, however rare, prolactinoma remains an important cause of male sexual dysfunction and infertility. Hypogonadism maybe the only manifestation of a macroprolactinoma in a male. This patient had a similar presentation without any local signs and symptoms. Secondly, hyperprolactinemia due to a macroprolactinoma may be a cause of reversible hypogonadotropic hypogonadism. Therefore, in the workup of male sexual dysfunction or infertility, serum prolactin assay should be routinely advised. Furthermore, in such a situation effective management of hyperprolactinemia/prolactinoma with dopamine agonists like cabergoline may restore eugonadism and fertility without the necessity of gonadal hormone replacement.

SUGGESTED READING

1. Melmed S, Kleinberg D. Williams Textbook of Endocrinology 13th edition. Philadelphia: Elsevier/Saunders; c2016. Chapter 9, Pituitary Masses and Tumors, Pages 232-99.

CASE 5: Secondary Hypothyroidism: Easy to Miss
Sudip Chatterjee

CASE HISTORY

A 49-year-old woman was seen on referral by a hematologist, to whom the patient had gone for a hemoglobin of 6.4 g/dL. She had swelling of her whole body for the last 6 months for which she was seeing a cardiologist. The patient had an extensive workup which did not show any major problem. Her ECG showed ST-T changes. Echocardiogram showed an ejection fraction of 54% with a chink of pericardial effusion. Urinalysis, urea creatinine and liver function tests were normal. TSH was 0.4 µU/mL. A diagnosis of dilated cardiomyopathy had been made and she was on furosemide, ranolazine digoxin nitrates and iron.

On examination, the patient had scanning speech, dry rough skin, and delayed relaxation of ankle jerks. She looked typically hypothyroid and hardly able to walk. The patient was admitted for further evaluation. A free T4 was requested which was grossly low at 0.2 ng/mL. A post Synacthen cortisol was 25.5 µg/dL (normal). Thyroxine was started in a dose of 25 µg per day and gradually increased by 25 µg every 2 weeks. MRI of the pituitary was normal. The patient was discharged and all her previous medicines were stopped.

Over the next 2 months, the patient had a dramatic improvement. All her symptoms resolved and she maintained a normal free T4 of 1.5 on 75 µg of thyroxine.

DISCUSSION

It is a common practice to check for hypothyroidism by ordering a TSH test alone. This often leads to mistakes as in this patient. Another related problem arises when a patient of secondary hypothyroidism is seen by a new physician. Here, TSH is invariably low as for example after pituitary surgery and the thyroxine dose is ofgten but incorrectly cut back leading to avoidable problems.

> **Take Home Messages**
>
> - The initial evaluation of thyroid function in a patient must always include T4 (preferably free T4) and TSH measurements. Merely measuring one of these values is not enough. When a patient of primary hypothyroidism is followed up over a period of time, TSH values alone may be used if there are cost considerations
> - In a patient with secondary hypothyroidism, TSH values are of no use in monitoring treatment. Here the target should be to keep the free T4 in the upper end of the normal range
> - Before treatment with thyroxine is started, an assessment should be made of the patient's cardiovascular risk. The risk is high in the elderly, in those with severe disease and in those with long-standing disease. In such situations, the dose of thyroxine should start low and go up in 25 µg increments every 2 weeks till the target dose is reached. In other situations, there is no need to step up the dose. For example in congenital hypothyroidism with a TSH of 100 µU/mL, there is no need to step up the dose. Similarly considerations apply in a patient who has recently turned hypothyroid after I-131 treatment for hyperthyroidism.

SUGGESTED READING

1. Gupta V, Lee M. Central hypothyroidism. Ind J Endocrinol Metab. 2011;15(Suppl 2):S99-106.
2. Koulouri O, Auldin MA, Agarwal R, et al. Diagnosis and treatment of hypothyroidism in TSH deficiency compared to primary thyroid disease: pituitary patients are at risk of under-replacement with levothyroxine. Clin Endocrinol (Oxf). 2011;74(6):744-9.

SECTION 12

Thyroid

CASE 1: Enlarged Pituitary in Primary Hypothyroidism
Ajitesh Roy

CASE HISTORY

A 15-year-old boy residing at South 24 Parganas, West Bengal, presented to Neurology OPD with a complaint of headache in occipital region and vertex for last 3 months. For the above said complaint a brain imaging was done which showed sellar mass. Patient was referred to endocrine OPD for further evaluation.

He was institutionally born at term through lower uterine segment Cesarean section from nonconsanguineous parents after an uncomplicated pregnancy. His neonatal period was uneventful and without having any history of birth asphyxia, prolonged jaundice or recurrent hypoglycemia.

He was noted to have arrest of growth and height for last 5 years for which his family did not seek any definite medical care. He also complained of increase sensitivity to cold, irregular bowel habits for several years. Parents also noted declining scholastic function and an inattentive behavior in him. Although they did not notice any mental retardation previously, and said that his development was normal until 10 years of age.

His parents were of normal height and stature. He did not complain of any diarrhea, vomiting, fever, recurrent infection, asthma and drug abuse. His past and family history was unremarkable.

On physical examination, his height was 143 cm (<3rd percentile) and weight 39 kg (<3rd percentile). Midparental height was within normal limit. Vitals—BP: 100/60 mm Hg, pulse rate: 72 beats/min. Pallor was present. There were hypertrichosis over his back (Figs. 1 and 2). Skin was dry. There was no goiter. Testes bilaterally palpable, normal in consistency, 4 mL (bilaterally). Pubic and axillary hair were sparse. Examination of other systems was unremarkable but ankle jerk was delayed. No other musculoskeletal abnormality was noted.

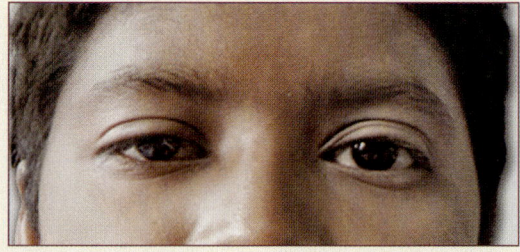

FIG. 1: Clinical stigma of hypothyroidism with congenital ptosisright eye.

MRI brain shows enlarged pituitary (13 mm × 12 mm × 11 mm) with diffuse enhancement with suprasellar extension. No obvious cortical lesion seen (Fig. 3). No focal SOL is separately visualized. The laboratory investigations are summarized in Table 1.

This patient was started on oral levothyroxine supplement initially at 100 μg/day and his TSH level dropped down to 1.14 μU/mL. A repeat MRI was done after 6 months which show marked regression in size of the pituitary. The gland was 6 mm × 7 mm × 9 mm in dimension (Fig. 4).

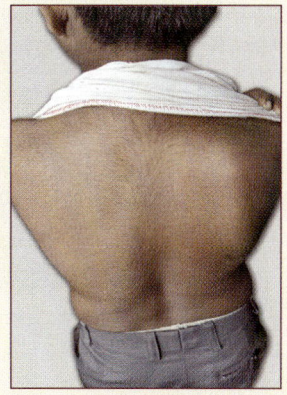

FIG. 2: Hypertrichosis at the back may be seen in hypothyroidism.

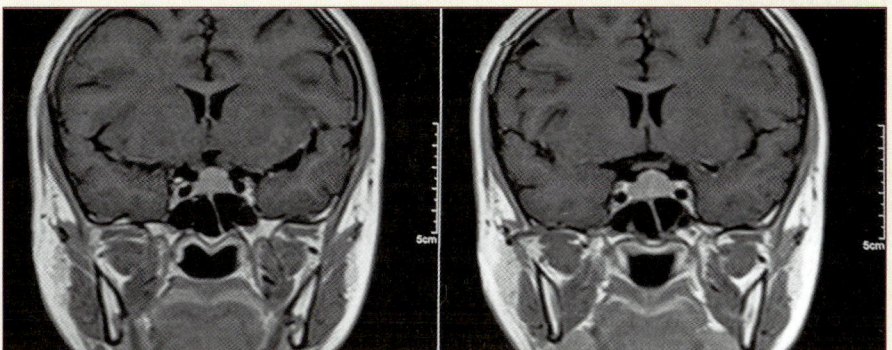

FIG. 3: Pre-treatment MRI (coronal section) of hypothalamo-pituitary region shows diffuse pituitary hyperplasia.

TABLE 1: Investigation.

Hemoglobin	9.8 g/dL, anisocytosis in RBC lineage
High-performance liquid chromatography	No hemoglobinopathy
Serum creatinine	1.1 mg/dL
Serum sodium	145 mmol/L
Serum potassium	4.8 mmol/L
Serum calcium	9.2 mg/dL
Liver function test	Normal
Albumin	4.9 g/dL
Globulin	3.8 g/dL
Urine RE	No abnormality detected
Insulin-like growth factor 1	159 ng/mL (237–996)
Prolactin	33.8 ng/mL (4.04–15.2)
TT4	<2 μg/dL (4.74–14.6)
Thyroid-stimulating hormone	>100 mIU/mL (0.53–3.59)
Anti-thyroid peroxidase	25 IU/mL (normal <35)
Anti-thyroglobulin	Not done

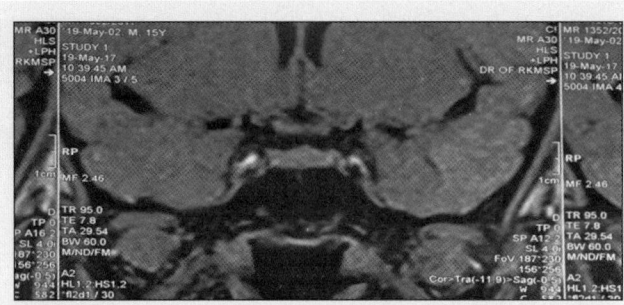

FIG. 4: Post-treatment MRI shows regression of size of pituitary.

DISCUSSION

Negative feedback from low thyroxine level leads to continuous stimulation of anterior pituitary enlargement due to overproduction of thyrotropin-releasing hormone (TRH) in primary hypothyroidism. TRH increases thyroid-stimulating hormone (TSH) from the pituitary gland in an attempt to elevate thyroxine levels to normal physiological levels; this long-standing hypothyroidism which is most commonly due to Hashimoto's thyroiditis causes hyperplasia of the pituitary's thyrotrophic cells. Usually there is no radiologically appreciable pituitary enlargement "in primary hypothyroidism". But after certain level, there starts a grossly visible anatomical change in the gland mostly leading to hyperplasia of the pituitary gland and sometimes adenoma causing symptoms of compression like headache and visual field defect.

There are many causes of sellar and suprasellar lesions. The differential diagnosis for a pituitary mass should include secondary enlargement from any endocrine end organ dysfunction, functioning or nonfunctioning pituitary adenoma and other lesions like craniopharyngioma, meningioma, etc. Primary hypothyroidism is one of the prototype examples of feedback adenoma, and it may even present with symptoms of elevated prolactin (PRL) levels with a pituitary mass. High PRL levels in such cases are due to the effect of TRH on lactotroph cells and it may also be attributed to compression of the infundibulum by the SOL.

Cases are reported where there is growth hormone deficiency in these patients though growth hormone axis should be evaluated after correction of hypothyroidism.

Secondary pituitary hyperplasia is often characterized by a homogeneously enhanced lesion on MRI which was evident in our case also. A trial of thyroxine replacement and repeat MRI after 12 weeks may help to correctly diagnose pituitary hyperplasia. Appropriate diagnosis and treatment are of utmost importance, as they can help avoid unnecessary treatment like surgery.

In our case, serum TSH and PRL levels started declining with thyroxine replacement. Surgery is reserved for decompression of the optic chiasm and optic nerve, or to obtain a tissue diagnosis in case the mass does not respond to thyroid hormone replacement. Our case showed a good response to thyroxine replacement; the post-contrast images also showed a regression in mass size, and the optic chiasm was free from the pituitary mass. If, in the course of follow-up with thyroid hormone replacement, the TSH levels partially decline and no improvement in the pituitary mass is seen, a diagnosis of TSH-secreting adenoma of the anterior pituitary must be considered and surgical resection is advised.

Section 12: Thyroid

> **Take Home Messages**
>
> - *Primary hypothyroidism presenting as a pituitary mass is a rare, but a well known entity so awareness of pituitary enlargement and the rare occurrence of neurologic symptoms are important in children with longstanding hypothyroidism*
> - *Recognition of this entity is crucial because complete regression can be achieved with thyroxine replacement therapy rather doing unnecessary pituitary surgery.*

SUGGESTED READING

1. Desai MP, Mehta RU, Choksi CS and Colaco MP. "Pituitary enlargement on magnetic resonance imaging in congenital hypothyroidism," Archives of Pediatrics and Adolescent Medicine. 1996;150(6):623-8.
2. Myers A, Hatanpaa K, Madden C, and Lingvay I, "Thyrotropin-secreting adenoma in a patient with primary hypothyroidism," Endocrine Practice. 2011;17(6):135–e139.
3. Nicholas WC, Russell WF. Primary hypothyroidism presenting as a pituitary mass. J Miss State Med Assoc. 2000;41:511-4.
4. Young M, Kattner K, Gupta K. Pituitary hyperplasia resulting from primary hypothyroidism mimicking macroadenomas. Br J Neurosurg. 1999;13:138-42.

CASE 2

Thyroid Ophthalmopathy

Sayan Ghosh, Somnath Raghuvanshi, Partha Sarathi Choudhury, Anirban Sinha, Animesh Maiti, Asish Kumar Basu

CASE HISTORY

A 57-year-old gentleman presented with bilateral eyelid swelling, proptosis and conjunctival congestion for last 8 months along with palpitation, tremors, hyperhidrosis and insomnia for last 1 year. He was diagnosed with diabetes mellitus 1 year back and was started on oral antidiabetic drugs. For last few months, his glycemic status was deteriorating. He was a chronic smoker (20 pack years) and was nonhypertensive.

TABLE 1: Investigations.	
Hemoglobin	13.5 g/dL
Total leukocyte count	5,670/mm^3
Differential leukocyte count	N67 L 26 E 2 M 5 B 0
Platelet	2.5 lac/mm^3
Serum creatinine	0.9 mg/dL
FPG/PPG	165 mg/dL/265 mg/dL
Chol/TG/HDL/LDL	149/120/55/79 mg/dL
SGOT/SGPT	56/50 IU/L
TSH/FT4	0.001 mIU/mL/4.25 ng/dL
2D ECHO	Normal study
LVEF	65%
Chest X-ray	WNL
ECG	Normal
CT orbit	Recti are bulky, retro-orbital fat planes are compressed, features suggestive of thyroid associated orbitopathy

Clinical examination: Pulse rate: 112 beats/min, blood pressure was 140/80 mm Hg, goiter grade 3, diffuse, acanthosis grade 1. Tremor present; no pretibial myxedema present.

Ophthalmologic examination: Bilateral exophthalmos present; clinical activity score (CAS): 3/7 (bilateral) (Fig. 1 and 2).

Diagnosis: Type 2 diabetes mellitus (T2DM) with Graves' disease with moderate to severe active thyroid associated orbitopathy (TAO).
- *In hospital course*: Carbimazole was started along with oral antidiabetic agents. He was treated with IV methylprednisolone weekly for 12 weeks (after achieving glycemic control) along with conservative management for thyroid associated orbitopathy.

  On follow-up, he became euthyroid and his hyperglycemia ameliorated; his liver enzymes normalized.

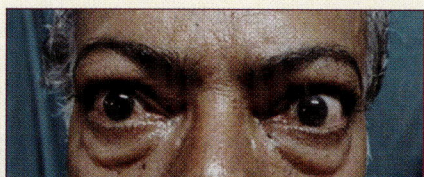

FIG. 1: Showing proptosis eye ball, lid-edema, conjunctival congestion.

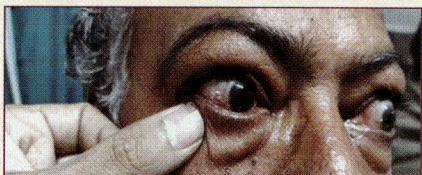

FIG. 2: Showing conjunctival edema.

DISCUSSION

Apart from the fact that Graves' disease may be associated with type 1 diabetes mellitus (T1DM), thyrotoxicosis due to Graves' disease may per se disturb the glucose tolerance in about one-third of patients with diabetes occurring in around 8% of them. There is evidence that insulin resistance is the underlying defect but insulin secretion is also disturbed. Excess thyroid hormones also increase hepatic glucose output.

Restoration of euthyroidism may improve the insulin resistance and hence amelioration of hyperglycemia. Even in insulin treated patients associated with hyperthyroidism, restoration of euthyroidism would lead to reduction of insulin requirement.

Take Home Message
- Graves' disease may coexist with type 2 diabetes or per se can lead to glucose intolerance. Restoration of euthyroidism in these patients could easily improve their glycemic control.

SUGGESTED READING

1. DeGroot's Text book of Endocrinology. 7th edition.
2. Harrison's Text book of Internal Medicine.19th edition. November 2014.
3. Melmed S, Polonsky KS, Larsen PR, Kronenberg HM. William's Text book of Endocrinology. 13th edition. January 2016.

CASE 3: Graves' Disease with Ocular Myasthenia Gravis

Anirban Mazumdar

CASE HISTORY

A 16-year-old female presented with weight loss, tremulousness of hands, and occasional palpitation for last 7 months. She had noticed a swelling in the anterior neck for the past 2 months. She had drooping of both eyelids for the past 20 days. There was some improvement in drooping of eyelids immediately after getting up from sleep. She also had oligomenorrhea for the past 9 months. She had no past history of thyroid or any autoimmune disorder in her first-degree relatives.

On examination, she was afebrile, had a thin build [body mass index (BMI) 17.8 kg/m^2], tachycardia (120 beats/min) and normal blood pressure. There was a grade 2 diffuse nontender soft palpable goiter without any associated bruit. Respiratory and cardiovascular system examination revealed no abnormality. Neurological examination revealed the presence of bilateral symmetrical fine tremor of hands and bilateral ptosis with incomplete external ophthalmoplegia. Pupillary size, shape, response and fundoscopy examination were normal. There was no evidence of any weakness in any other muscle group or any signs of bulbar muscle weakness. Biochemical investigation are summarized in Table 1.

TABLE 1: Biochemical investigation.

Tests	Value	Normal range
Fasting plasma glucose	90 mg/dL	70–99
Serum creatinine	0.66 mg/dL	0.6–1.2
Prolactin	14.60 ng/mL	4–30
Follicle-stimulating hormone	5.3 mIU/mL	2–12
Luteinizing hormone	2.2 mIU/mL	1–18
Thyroid function tests		
Free T3	8.16 pg/mL	2.50–5.50
Free T4	4.11 ng/dL	0.85–1.80
Thyroid-stimulating hormone	<0.001	0.50–5.50

Anti-thyroid peroxidase antibody and TSH receptor antibody (TRAb) were strongly positive. Ultrasonography (USG) of thyroid gland revealed diffuse enlargement with increased intrathyroidal vascularity. Hematological parameters and liver function tests were normal. The Technetium-99m (Tc-99m) thyroid scan showed diffuse increased tracer activity of the gland suggestive of hyperfunctioning of the gland. CT scan of the orbit did not show any evidence of proptosis or extraocular muscle thickening. MRI scan of brain was normal. Repetitive nerve stimulation test (RNST) of both facial nerves, right ulnar nerve, and left spinal accessory nerve showed no significant decremental response on stimulation. However, anti-acetylcholine receptor antibody (anti-AchR Ab) titer was elevated 4.34 nmol/L (normal: <0.5 nmol/L). High resolution computerized tomography without contrast of thorax revealed the presence of a mildly enlarged thymus. The patient showed significant improvement in ptosis and external ophthalmoplegia 1 hour after neostigmine (0.5 mg/1 mL) intramuscular injection (Figs. 1–3) and revealed the characteristic upper eyelid retraction sign of Graves' ophthalmopathy (predominantly on right side). Based on the above findings a diagnosis of Graves' disease (GD) with ocular myasthenia gravis (OMG) was made.

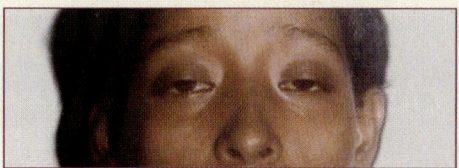

FIG. 1: Before neostigmine.

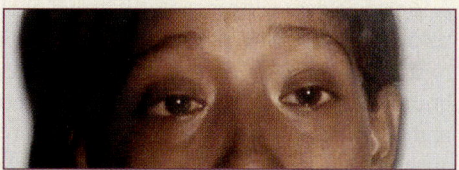

FIG. 2: 30 minutes after neostigmine.

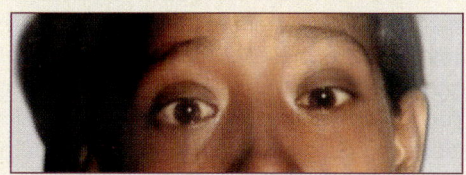

FIG. 3: 60 minutes after neostigmine.

The patient was prescribed carbimazole 30 mg daily for GD and pyridostigmine (60 mg) thrice daily for OMG. On a 2-month follow-up, the patient showed considerable improvement in physical and biochemical parameters of thyrotoxicosis and significant improvement in OMG with mild residual ptosis and minimal ophthalmoplegia.

DISCUSSION

Graves' disease is an autoimmune thyroid disease (AITD) and is the most common cause of thyrotoxicosis. Ophthalmopathy is one of the striking features of GD, present in almost 20% of GD and at times is the sole presenting feature. GD is associated with various autoimmune disorders, such as myasthenia gravis (MG), type 1 diabetes mellitus, pernicious anemia, and autoimmune adrenal insufficiency. MG is reported in a fairly low frequency (0.2%) of patients with AITD. Usually a milder form of OMG is associated with AITD. Patients with OMG and GD usually do not develop the generalized form of MG. The higher frequency of ocular MG in AITD could be that these disorders have a common genetic background. In most patients with both GD and OMG, thyrotoxic symptoms occur before or concurrently with those of myasthenia. Treatment of thyroid disorder in patients with MG leads to myasthenia regression in approximately two-thirds of the patients. The ocular changes in GD may include lid retraction, lid lag, exophthalmos, periorbital edema, chemosis and ophthalmoplegia (mostly the superior and lateral recti). All these signs are often obscured by the presence of ptosis from OMG as demonstrated in this case.

Myasthenia gravis has a high incidence (5–10%) in patients with GD and other autoimmune thyroid diseases. Interestingly, 40% people with OMG have anti-thyroid antibodies. The most common lid feature of GD is lid reaction while that of ocular MG is ptosis. The signs of external ophthalmoplegia can occur due to infiltration of extraocular muscles as in GD or may be the sole manifestation of OMG. Hence, ophthalmoplegia may pose a significant diagnostic difficulty to the treating physician. The presence of ptosis is a robust clinical clue to the possibility of myasthenia. Orbicularis oculi weakness in combination with ptosis and external ophthalmoparesis is a strong indicator of OMG. Thus patients with OMG who are presented with lid retraction or GD who are presented with ptosis should be considered to have both disorders.

Repetitive nerve stimulation studies (RNST) and single-fiber electromyography (SFEMG) are recommended in the diagnosis of MG. The decremental response of muscle action potential amplitude in RNST is seen in only 33% of patients with purely OMG. SFEMG has a sensitive of 85–100% for OMG when used on the frontalis or orbicularis oculi muscle and a sensitivity of 91–100% in generalized MG. Antibody tests (anti-AChR antibodies) are also less sensitive (positive in only 50%) is patients with OMG (versus 80–99% in generalized MG). Acetylcholinesterase inhibitor test (infusion of IV edrophonium chloride) is a highly sensitive test for generalized MG and OMG but is not routinely done because of adverse consequences. The test is most useful to demonstrate improvement in ptosis or in extraocular muscle motility. Neostigmine stimulation is safe method to diagnose cases of OM and MG with ocular involvement.

Fifty percent of patients presenting with OMG develop generalized weakness within 6 months and 80% within 2 years. Patients with OMG without any progression for 2 years are likely to have symptoms restricted to the ocular muscles thereafter. MG is commonly treated with anticholinesterase medications supplemented by immunosuppression, plasmapheresis and/or thymectomy. Management of thyroid dysfunction often alleviates the myasthenic symptoms and achieving and maintaining euthyroid status is of paramount importance when both disorders are present concomitantly. Enlarged thymus may be present in both disorders and early thymectomy may have potential beneficial effect on MG.

Take Home Message
- *Importance of detecting coexisting OMG in patient with GD.*

SUGGESTED READING

1. Akau M. Complete Bilateral External Ophthalmoplegia: OMG a 'Grave' Diagnosis. [online] Available from https://www.aaopt.org/docs/knowledge-base/melanie-akau.pdf?sfvrsn=3f488609_0. [Last accessed June, 2019].
2. Kubiszewska J, Szyluk B, Szczudlik P, et al. Prevalence and impact of autoimmune thyroid disease on myasthenia gravis course. Brain Behav. 2016;6(10):e00537. [online] Available from https://doi.org/10.1002/brb3.537. [Last accessed June, 2019].
3. Nair AG, Patil-Chhablani P, Venkatramani DV, et al. Ocular myasthenia gravis: a review. Indian J Ophthalmol. 2014;62:985-91.

CASE 4
Gestational Thyrotoxicosis
Binayak Sinha

CASE HISTORY

A 24-year-old lady who was 8 weeks pregnant had been seeing her obstetrician regularly since conception with nausea and vomiting. This was her first pregnancy. She had recently complained of worsening malaise and palpitations. The obstetrician had requested some routine tests including a complete blood count, renal and liver function tests, fasting plasma glucose, thyroid function tests and some routine tests of urine and stools. An abdominal ultrasound had also been sought.

The tests turned out to be all completely within normal limits except for the thyroid function which showed a thyroid-stimulating hormone (TSH) suppressed at less than 0.001 mIU/L (Normal: 0.3–4.5 mIU/L) with a total T4 14 µg/dL (Normal: 4.6–12 µg/dL) and a total T3 of 259 ng/dL (Normal: 80–180 ng/dL).

She was referred to the endocrinologist who noted that this lady had no history of thyroid disease and except for the nausea vomiting and palpitations had noted a weight loss of 2 kg in the last 2 months. Her periods had been regular and she had no previous history of note. She had no addictions. Clinical examination revealed a heart rate of 112 beats/min, with a blood pressure of 110/70 mm Hg. She had no goiter but had fine tremor of her hands. Her eyes were normal with no signs of exophthalmos.
A diagnosis of thyrotoxicosis was made.

PHYSIOLOGIC CHANGES OF THYROID FUNCTION IN PREGNANCY

During the first trimester of pregnancy, hCG (human chorionic gonadotropin) levels spike as conception occurs and this concurrently stimulates the TSH receptors which have a structural similarity. Along with this elevated levels of estrogen lead to a rise in thyroid-binding globulin (TBG). These changes translate into a suppression of TSH levels initially which normalize by the second trimester. Alongside a suppression of TSH total T4 levels are elevated initially, normalizing by the end of the second trimester. There is minimal change in free T4 or free T3 levels.

DIFFERENTIAL DIAGNOSIS OF THYROTOXICOSIS DIAGNOSED IN PREGNANCY

All forms of hyperthyroidism including Graves' disease, multinodular goiter and solitary toxic nodule and subacute thyroiditis may present in pregnancy. However, the main differential of these inherent thyroid disorders is gestational thyrotoxicosis which presents in the first trimester of pregnancy and is associated with significant nausea and vomiting usually. In fact, it is often associated with hyperemesis gravidarum. It is extremely important to make a correct diagnosis as gestational thyrotoxicosis is self-limiting and resolves by itself at the end of the first trimester when the hCG levels begin to plateau and the nausea and vomiting ceases to be a concern for most women.

Since imaging with ionizing radiation is contraindicated in pregnancy, the best way to differentiate Graves' disease from gestational thyrotoxicosis is by testing for TSH receptor antibody (TRAb). A positive TRAb indicates Graves' disease. A negative TRAb in association with a normal ultrasonography of the thyroid gland is almost diagnostic of gestational thyrotoxicosis.

MANAGEMENT OF THYROTOXICOSIS IN PREGNANCY

Gestational thyrotoxicosis is a self-limiting disorder and is usually managed with antiemetics and β-blockers. TSH values should be monitored to ensure normalization.

If however Graves' disease is diagnosed in the first trimester, propylthiouracil (PTU) should be started. Thyroid function should be monitored every 6 weeks with measurement of TSH and free T4 and T3 levels. Falling titers of TRAB are indicative of improvement. Methimazole or carbimazole may be used for treatment of Graves' disease in the second trimester. The lowest possible dose of either group of drugs should be used.

Inadequate response to antithyroid drugs in pregnancy is an indication for thyroidectomy and surgery may be performed electively in the second trimester, if necessary.

There is no role of radioactive iodine during pregnancy. Ultrasound of the thyroid revealed no abnormality and TRAb was negative. She was put onto antiemetics and propranolol 10 mg twice a day. She improved over the next month and her TSH level at the 13th week of gestation was 1.8 mIU/L. She, thereafter, had regular thyroid function tests through her pregnancy which remained completely normal. Her pregnancy followed an unremarkable course and she delivered a healthy child at 39 weeks gestation by elective cesarean section. The infant's TSH level was normal at birth. The mother has not been seen in the endocrine clinic thereafter.

DISCUSSION

All forms of thyroid disease may present in pregnancy. However thyrotoxicosis of pregnancy is an unique entity caused by the interactions of the pregnancy hormones with TSH. A careful history and measurement of TRAbs levels help to elict the diagnosis. Treatment is symptomatic.

> ### Take Home Messages
> - *Physicians must be aware of the diagnosis of gestational thyrotoxicosis which requires only symptomatic treatment and is self limiting*
> - *Occurring in the first trimester gestational thyrotoxicosis is associated with severe nausea and vomiting*
> - *A negative TSH receptor antibody level (TRAb) indicates a diagnosis of gestational thyrotoxicosis*
> - *However the physician must also be aware that all other forms of thyrotoxicosis may present in pregnancy and use adequate measures to make a correct diagnosis prior to starting treatment for this condition.*

SUGGESTED READING

1. Baidya B, Pearce S. Diagnosis and management of thyrotoxicosis. BMJ. 2014;349:g5128.
2. Reid J, Wheeler S. Hyperthyroidism: diagnosis and treatment. Am Fam Physician. 2005;72:623-30, 635-6.
3. Ross D, Burch H, Cooper D, et al. 2016 American Thyroid Association Guidelines for Diagnosis and Management of Hyperthyroidism and Other Causes of Thyrotoxicosis. Thyroid. 2016;26(10):1343-421.

CASE 5
A Case of Thyrotoxic Periodic Paralysis due to Painless Thyroiditis*

Debmalya Sanyal

CASE HISTORY

A 20-year-old male presented with sudden onset flaccid quadriparesis with no preceding history of fever, dysphagia, dysphonia, diplopia, bladder, or bowel involvement. There was no relation with heavy carbohydrate meal, exercise or diarrhea, and no past history of similar episode. Examination revealed lower limb proximal muscle power of 3/5, diminished deep tendon reflexes (DTR) in all four limbs, bilateral flexor plantar responses, no cranial nerve palsy and no respiratory muscle involvement. Goiter and clinical feature of thyrotoxicosis were absent. Serum potassium was 2.2 mmol/L (normal: 3.5–5) and ESR: 38 mm/h (normal: 1–25). Thyroid function tests (TFT) showed, free T4 2.4 ng/dL (normal: 0.7–2.0), TSH : 0.06 (normal: 0.5-5), and TPO antibody 54 IU/mL (normal). Technetium-99m (^{99m}Tc) pertechnetate thyroid scan revealed decreased uptake: 0.1% (nl. 0.4–1%) consistent with thyroiditis. Thyroid FNAC found features suggestive of thyroiditis (lymphocytic infiltration, no giant cells). EMG showed myopathic pattern, no decremental muscle action potential.

DISCUSSION

Thyrotoxic periodic paralysis (TPP) is a rare disorder characterized by episodic muscle weakness due to hypokalemia with delayed diagnosis due to subtleness of the clinical features of thyrotoxicosis differentiating from familial hypokalemic periodic paralysis (FHPP) may be difficult (Table 1). Many patients of TPP may not have obvious signs and symptoms of thyrotoxicosis, as seen in our case of painless thyroiditis. In TPP, involvement is mostly proximal and motor resulting in quadriparesis without bowel and bladder affection as in our case. Impairment of bulbar or respiratory muscles is rare. Hypokalemia of less than 3.0 mmol/L is the hallmark of TPP and the degree of initial hypokalemia has a direct correlation with the severity of paralysis but not with the thyroid

TABLE 1: Comparison between thyrotoxic periodic paralysis (TPP) and familial hypokalemic periodic paralysis (FHPP).

TPP	FHPP
<20 years	20–40 years
Predominantly male	Equal sex distribution
Sporadic	Autosomal dominant
Asian, Indian/Hispanic	Caucasian, Asian
History of thyrotoxicosis	History of hypokalemic paralysis
Clinical features of hyperthyroidism present	Clinical features of hyperthyroidism absent

---

With permission from: Sanyal D, Raychaudhuri M, Bhattacharjee S. Three cases of thyrotoxic periodic paralysis due to painless thyroiditis. Indian J Endocrinol Metab. 2013;17(Suppl 1):S162-3.

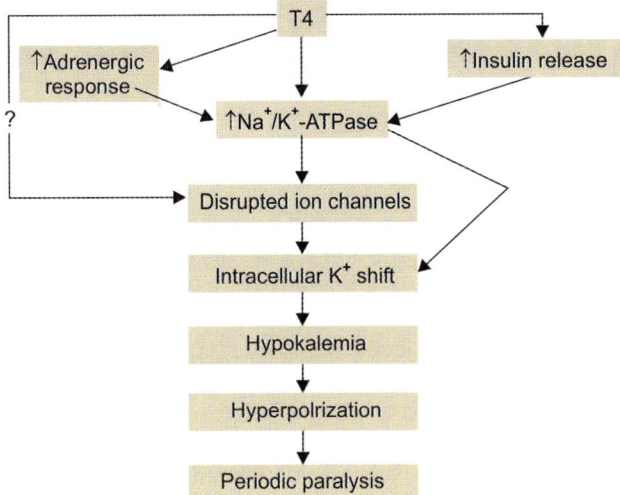

FLOWCHART 1: Mechanisms for muscle weakness in thyrotoxic periodic paralysis.

hormone level. Hypokalemia is most likely due to high levels of thyroid hormone causing overactivity of the Na^+-K^+-ATPase pump triggering intracellular shift of the potassium causing muscle hyperpolarization vide (Flowchart 1). In cases of acute attacks of TPP, immediate restoration of serum potassium via intravenous route and oral propranolol is necessary. Because TPP does not recur once the patient is euthyroid, adequate control of hyperthyroidism by antithyroid drugs, radioiodine therapy or thyroidectomy is imperative. β-adrenergic blockers like propranolol prevent attacks until euthyroidism is achieved.

CONCLUSION

Quadriparesis due to TPP may be the presenting feature of thyrotoxicosis of any etiology including painless thyroiditis. The painless nature of thyroiditis and absence of clinical signs of thyrotoxicosis can delay diagnosis and treatment. Routine evaluation of thyroid function assay in patients with hypokalemic paralysis is necessary to distinguish TPP from other forms of hypokalemic paralysis.

> **Take Home Message**
>
> - *TPP can a rare presenting feature of all forms thyrotoxicosis, though overt manifestation of thyrotoxicosis may be absent.*

SUGGESTED READING

1. Kung AW. Thyrotoxic periodic paralysis: A diagnostic challenge. J Clin Endocrinol Metab 2006;91:2490-5.
2. Tinker TD, Vannatta JB. Thyrotoxic hypokalemic periodic paralysis: Report of four cases and review of the literature. J Okla State Med Assoc 1987;80:76-83.

CASE 6: Myxedema Coma: Rare but Dangerous

Soumyabrata Roy Chaudhuri

CASE HISTORY

A 92-year-old male, hypertensive, hypothyroid, chronic kidney disease (CKD) with serum creatinine ranging between 2 mg/dL and 2.5 mg/dL, on a permanent pacemaker for recurrent syncope for last 7 years was admitted to hospital with decreasing urine output and massive fluid overload. There were no signs of infection either in the urine or in the blood culture sent. The total leukocyte count (TLC), c-reactive protein (CRP) were also normal, albumin was 2.1 g/dL, urea was 37.87 mg/dL and serum creatinine was 3.86 mg/dL. Nephrologist advised albumin infusion with infusion of furosemide and fluid restriction to the tune of 800 mL/24 hours for 3 days. Even on day 4 there was no significant diuresis to enable the patient to be offloaded. The Nephrologist discussed pros and cons of sustained low efficiency dialysis (SLED) with his two sons and slated him for alternate day SLED with an ultrafiltration of 3 L/day. However after the third and fourth session of SLED patient became confused agitated and then stuporous. He began to desaturate with a pulse oximeter reading O_2 saturation of 65–75% in room air and requiring 4 L of oxygen support to keep O_2 saturation above 92% ABG read pH 7.41, pCO_2: 63 mm Hg, pO_2: 42%, HCO_3: 33.6 mmol/L, BE: 7.8 mmol/L, O_2 saturation 74%. Body temperature was between 98.5–97°F.

Mr SMC was shifted to intensive care and a bi-PAP support was started. Chest X-ray showed bilateral pleural effusion and fresh infiltrates. A sample of pleural aspirate was sent for culture and sensitivity which later on came out to be sterile. Serum sodium was 122 mEq/L and potassium was 2.9 mEq/L (despite the fact that the patient was receiving SLED on alternate days) and CRP jumped from 17 to 139. Antibiotics were uptitrated and a Ryle's tube was inserted. Thyroid-stimulating hormone (TSH) sprung a surprise; it was recorded values as greater than 100 U/dL although Mr SMC was receiving a levothyroxine supplement of 50 μg for a long time with stable thyroid function tests done at recommended intervals. A blood sample for random cortisol was sent and hydrocortisone was started via intravenous access at a dose of 50 mg × 6 hourly and 300 μg of levothyroxine was given as a loading dose via Ryle's tube and then 100 μg was continued daily. TSH came down to 31.22 U/dL 4 days after the loading dose of administration. As random cortisol came out to be normal steroid was withdrawn after day 5. Meanwhile his infective parameters settled and CRP gradually reduced to 20. He was weaned off bi-PAP support and gradually weaned off oxygen support too. TSH remained stable at the same range on day 14 after the loading dose. As the vascular access was difficult in terms of an AV fistula due to poor blood flow a permanent catheter was implanted via the left subclavian route. He was discharged with the permanent catheter and is well on two sessions of hemodialysis done at a nearby center on an OPD basis. Date wise summary of in-hospital investigation is provided in the Tables 1, 2, and 3 which follow.

Section 12: Thyroid

TABLE 1: Datewise in-hospital investigation report.

Date	Medical Test Report							Name: SMC Age: 92 years			
	Serum sodium	Serum potassium	Uric acid	Serum creatinine	Glucose	Urea	BUN	Hemoglobin	C-reactive protein (CRP)	TSH
Normal range	136–149 mEq/dL	3.8–5.2 mEq/dL	3.5–7.2 mg/dL	0.66–1.25 mg/dL	70–100 mg/dL	17–43 mg/dL	9–20	13–18 g/dL	<10	0.27–4.2 U/dL
28-Jan-19	131.00	3.80		3.86		37.57			5.00	
28-Jan-19								10.50		
30-Jan-19		3.90		3.91		39.62				
3-Feb-19	133.00	3.00		2.33		21.86		8.60	19.80	
4-Feb-19	132.00	2.90		1.63		13.17		8.60	23.40	
8-Feb-19	127.00	2.70		1.22		10.22		10.30	17.80	
13-Feb-19								9.90		>100
17-Feb-19	120.00	3.00		1.74		36.45			139.90	
19-Feb-19	122.00	3.50		1.73		48.33			88	31.22
22-Feb-19	126.00	3.80		1.07		34.47			56	
24-Feb-19	130.00	2.50		2.51		81.49				
26-Feb-19	133.00	2.60		2.14		54.40		8.00		35.29
1-Mar-19	135.00	3.30							20.00	
5-Mar-19	136.00	4.50		2.71		84.00			5.00	

(TSH: thyroid stimulating hormone)

TABLE 2: Datewise in-hospital investigation reports.

Date	SGOT	SGPT	Total protein	Albumin
Normal range	17–59 U/L	21–72 U/L	6.3–8.2 G/DL	3.5–5.0 G/DL
28-Jan-19	22.00	23.00	5.80	2.40
29-Jan-19				
30-Jan-19				2.30
31-Jan-19				
3-Feb-19				
3-Feb-19				
6-Feb-19				
8-Feb-19				2.60
11-Feb-19				3.00
14-Feb-19	24.00	24.00	6.20	3.10
22-Feb-19				3.20

(SGOT: serum glutamic-oxaloacetic transaminase; SGPT: serum glutamic-pyruvic transaminase)

TABLE 3: Datewise in-hospital investigation reports.

Date	Total leukocyte count	Neutrophil
Normal range	4,000–10,000/mm^3	40–80%
28-Jan-19	4,700.00	75.00
3-Feb-19	4,500.00	71.00
4-Feb-19	5,000.00	77.00
8-Feb-19	4,200.00	79.00
11-Feb-19		
13-Feb-19	5,300.00	82.00
17-Feb-19		
19-Feb-19	16,500.00	94.00
22-Feb-19	8,900.00	86.00
26-Feb-19	8,200.00	85.00
1-Mar-19	8,900.00	83.00
5-Mar-19	5,600.00	73.00

DISCUSSION

Myxedema coma, the extreme expression of hypothyroidism, is a medical emergency requiring a high degree of clinical suspicion. The term myxedema was proposed by Ord in 1878 to describe the peculiar nonpitting swelling of skin in the hypothyroid adult and has been used interchangeably with hypothyroidism in the medical literature. Although

TABLE 4: Diagnostic scoring system for myxedema coma.*

Thermoregulatory dysfunction (Temperature °F/°C)	Points
>95/35	0
89.6–95/32–35	10
<89.6/32	20
• Central nervous system effects	
○ Absent	0
○ Somnolent/Lethargy	10
○ Obtunded	15
○ Stupor	20
○ Coma/seizures	30
• Gastrointestinal findings	
○ Anorexia/abdominal pain/constipation	5
○ Decreased intestinal motility	15
○ Paralytic ileus	20
• Precipitating event	
○ Absent	0
○ Present	10
• Cardiovascular dysfunction	
○ Bradycardia/heart rate	
− Absent	0
− 50–59	10
− 40–49	20
− <40	30
○ Other ECG changes**	10
− Pericardial/pleural effusion	10
− Pulmonary edema	15
− Cardiomegaly	15
− Hypotension	20
• Metabolic disturbances	
○ Hyponatremia	10
○ Hypoglycemia	10
○ Hypoxemia	10
○ Hypercarbia	10
○ Decrease in GFR	10

*Adapted from Popoveniuc G, ChaNdra T, Sud A, et al. A diagnostic scoring system for myxedema coma. Endocr Pract. 2014;20(8)808-17.
**Other EKG changes: QT prolongation, or low voltage complex, or bundle branch blocks, or nonspecific ST-T changes, or heart blocks.

Note: Total score: >60 highly suggestive/diagnostic of myxedema coma
25–59 supportive of diagnosis of myxedema coma
<25 myxedema coma unlikely.

the actual incidence is unknown, myxedema coma is uncommon, only 200 cases were reported between 1953 and 1986. The mortality rate in these patients is 50% or greater even with immediate thyroid hormone replacement therapy and supportive measures. Early recognition and intervention can be lifesaving.

Myxedema coma occurs almost exclusively during or after the sixth decade with 80% of the cases occurring in women. More than 90% of cases have been reported to have occurred during winter months and are frequently associated with intercurrent illness like pneumonia or other infections. Sedating drugs are also common precipitants. About a half of myxedema coma patients do lapse into coma after admission to the hospital, probably as the result of stress caused by diagnostic and therapeutic interventions encountered during hospitalization.

A scoring system has made life easier for us, clinicians to diagnose myxedema crisis with a greater degree of accuracy. Mr SMC here, for example, had a score of 75 and thus there was no diagnostic dilemma (stupor: 20, constipation: 5, precipitating event: 10, pleural effusion: 10, hypoxemia: 10, hypercarbia: 10, decrease in GFR: 10). In this case due to presence of permanent pacemaker bradycardia was not recorded and due to ongoing SLED hyponatremia was partially corrected and so these two cardinal features could not be seen at the expected levels. Hence in elderly hypothyroid subjects myxedema coma is a differential diagnosis that should not be missed out even if septic metabolic encephalopathy is much more common.

Take Home Message

- *In case of acute confusional state especially in elderly subjects with history of hypothyroidism myxedema crisis is a possibility to explore in addition to commoner diagnoses like septic/metabolic encephalopathy.*

SUGGESTED READING

1. American Thyroid Association. Clinical Thyroidology for the Public: A publication of the American Thyroid Association. Summaries for the Public from recent articles in Clinical Thyroidology. 2017;10(4):3-4.
2. Kim MI. Hypothyroidism in the Elderly. 2017.
3. Mathew V, Misgar RA, Ghosh S, et al. Myxedema Coma: A New Look into an Old Crisis. J Thyroid Res. 2011;2011:493462.
4. Olsen CG. Myxedema coma in the elderly. J Am Board Fam Pract. 1995;8:376-83.

CASE 7: An Unusual Patient with Thyroiditis
Sudip Chatterjee

CASE HISTORY

Mr SS, a 44-year-old man was first seen in May 2000. He had been suffering from hyperthyroid from 1997 and had been on carbimazole for 3 years but relapsed on stopping. He was given 5 mCi of I-131 in 2000. He became euthyroid but relapsed after 1 year. Carbimazole was restarted but again relapsed after stopping and then he had another dose of I-131 in 2004. Three months later he became and was started on thyroxine. Meanwhile, the patient got a job in the State Education Department, married and had a girl. He was not on follow-up from 2004–2010. He stopped thyroxine on his own in 2010 and thyroid-stimulating hormone (TSH) rose to 42.4 µU/mL. He then came for a consultation in 2010. He remained euthyroid on 50 µg thyroxine till June 2012, when he presented with hyperthyroidism. At that time he also had fever and thyroid tenderness and was thought to have subacute thyroiditis (SAT). There was no way of proving the diagnosis as the patient was on thyroxine. Thyroxine was stopped and the free T4 came down from 3.7 to 2.2, but was still high. Eventually the patient became hypothyroid and was put back on thyroxine. On looking back, there seemed to be a similar attack of SAT in 2008 for which he consulted elsewhere. In June 2014, there was another attack of SAT. By now the patient could recognize the symptoms, stop his thyroxine and restart later. He had another episode in July 2016. This time the patient stopped thyroxine on his own, but developed paroxysmal atrial fibrillation.

It was decided to permanently ablate the thyroid when the opportunity presented itself. In the recovery phase of SAT, there is usually increased iodine uptake by the thyroid as the gland tries to repair itself. After this fourth episode of SAT, a thyroid scan was requested every 6 weeks. After 12 weeks, there was a dense picture and the patient was given 8 mCi of I-131. Figures 1–3 show the changing nature of the Tc99 thyroid scan of this patient during the acute, early recovery and late recovery stage of the fourth episode of thyroiditis of this patient. By October 2017, the patient was hypothyroid and well replaced on 100 µg thyroxine. The patient was last seen in October 2018, and was doing well.

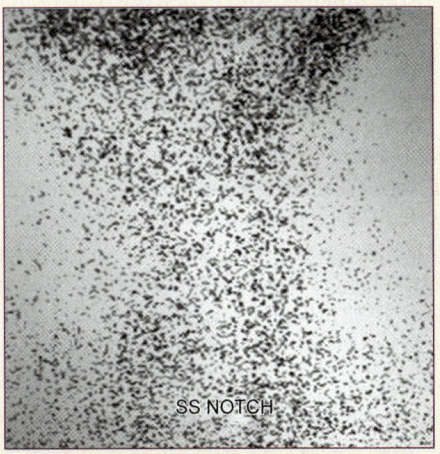

FIG. 1: Technetium-99m (Tc-99m) thyroid scan of SS showing subacute thyroiditis (SAT). Fourth episode in July 2016.

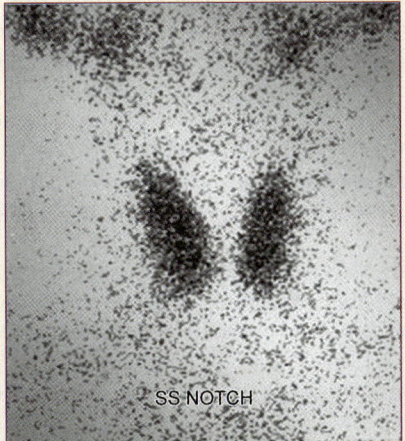

FIG. 2: Technetium-99m (Tc-99m) scan of Mr SS after 6 weeks showing patchy uptake of the radioisotope. Fourth episode, continuing.

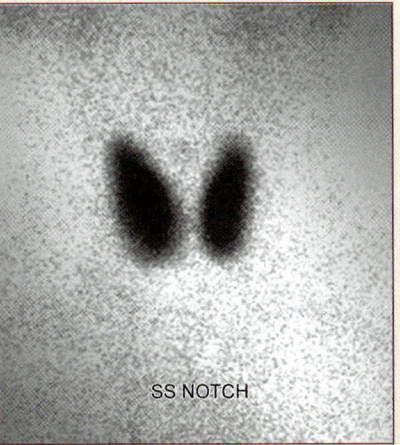

FIG. 3: Technetium-99m (Tc-99m) scan of Mr SS after 10 weeks, showing a dense pattern. Same episode just before I-131 was administered.

DISCUSSION

All patients of hyperthyroidism do not have Graves' disease warranting treatment with carbimazole. This patient was unusual in that in his case Graves' hyperthyroidism was followed by episodes of thyroiditis. It is imperative that a Technetium-99m scan be done. In thyroiditis, as also in excessive iodine intake and in thyroiditis factitia (surreptitious intake of thyroxine) the scan will show no uptake by the thyroid gland while there will be visible uptake by the salivary glands. In hyperthyroidism by contrast, there will be a dense uptake of the radio pharmaceutical by the thyroid leaving no isotope to be taken up by the salivary gland. A typical dose is 1–2 mCi. Although not advised, there have been instances where this dose has been given in pregnancy without adverse effects to the fetus. This patient illustrates the critical role the thyroid scan played in diagnosis and treatment. Initially the patient had hyperthyroidism treated with carbimazole and finally I-131. Later, the patient went on to have four episodes of subacute thyroiditis. Three episodes were documented and in one the patient made the diagnosis himself. A scan done while a patient is on thyroxine is not helpful as in no case will there be uptake by the thyroid. Thus subacute thyroiditis in a patient already taking thyroxine can only be done on the basis of a history and clinical suspicion.

In the acute phase, treatment is with paracetamol and NSAIDs. Antibiotics do not have a role to play. In severe cases where the gland is tender to touch, low doses of prednisolone may be given. This causes quick resolution of symptoms, which however tend to recur when the drug is withdrawn.

Mr SS did not need glucocorticoids on any occasion. We were forced to act when the fourth episode was complicated by atrial fibrillation. Treatment with a strategically timed dose of I-131 to ablate residual thyroid tissue has been used before. This treatment turned out to be very effective as the patient has remained well ever since.

Take Home Messages

- *Subacute or de Quervain's thyroiditis is a fairly common condition. It is generally thought to be due to a viral infection and is associated with fever and upper respiratory infection. Autoimmune and HLA associations have been noted. In the initial stage there is hyperthyroidism due to destruction of the thyroid follicles and release of stored thyroid hormone into the circulation. This is spontaneously followed by euthyroidism after which there is a prolonged hypothyroid phase during which the gland recovers from the damage*
- *In the initial phase the Technetium 99m pertechnetate scan characteristically does not visualize the thyroid and there may be more uptake of the isotope in the salivary glands. The appearance of the scan changes with time and in the recovery phase there can be a dense picture of the thyroid similar to that seen in Graves' disease (but without hyperthyroidism)*
- *There is no fixed time course for the changes in the scanned images to occur. In this patient it took 10 weeks from the second scan to get a dense picture of the thyroid as seen in the third scan*
- *As SAT is a benign and self-limiting condition, active treatment is not advised after the acute phase is over except for temporary thyroxine support in the hypothyroid phase. This patient had four attacks and the last attack was associated with a potentially dangerous condition, i.e. atrial fibrillation*
- *It was therefore decided to take advantage of the "dense stage" and administer an ablative dose of I-131.*

SUGGESTED READING

1. Kitchener MI, Chapman IM. Subacute thyroiditis: a review of 105 cases. Clin Nucl Med. 1989;14(6): 439-42.
2. Volpé R. The management of subacute (DeQuervain's) thyroiditis. Thyroid. 1993;3(3):253-5.
3. Wartofsky L. Radioiodine therapy for Graves' disease: case selection and restrictions recommended to patients in North America. Thyroid. 1997;7(2):213-6.

CASE 8: A Hyperthyroid Child

Sudip Chatterjee

CASE HISTORY

A 24-year-old female was seen in 2007 when she was 11 years old. She had hyperthyroidism with a 10-g goiter and lid retraction. Thyroid-stimulating hormone (TSH) receptor antibody was positive. Carbimazole was started and she and her parents were counseled about I-131 treatment. She had some behavioral problems and needed counseling. The patient was well-controlled and lid retraction normalized. In 2009, it was suggested that carbimazole should be stopped and I-131 could be used if there was a relapse. The parents declined and did not return for 2 years. The patient's mother came in 2011 because she developed hypothyroidism. They were now willing to consider I-131. Carbimazole was stopped hyperthyroidism reappeared. She was given 5 mCi of I-131 in May 2011. She became hypothyroid in September 2011 and has been doing well on thyroxine ever since.

Review of clinic data from 1996 to 2019 showed 127 patients with hyperthyroidism in the age group 3–18 years. 79% were female and 95% had Graves' disease. The calculated remission rate was 21%, based on incomplete data. This is because 51% of patients dropped out of follow-up when I-131 was discussed. I-131 treatment was accepted by only 2 patients. Remission rates in children are as low as 20–30% on carbimazole. Treatment beyond 18 months is unlikely to improve the remission rate.

There are extensive data to show that I-131 treatment for hyperthyroidism is devoid of long-term sequelae. There is no contraindication to use it after 10 years of age. It has no effect on future malignancy or infertility. However women taking I-131 are advised to avoid pregnancy for 1 year and men for 6 months. There are major cultural differences surrounding the acceptability of I-131. For example, it is accepted by 60% of patients as the first modality of treatment in the US versus 0% in Japan.

The patient described here is typical of series of patients published by us, and documents the difficulty in treating young hyperthyroid patients.

DISCUSSION

This patient illustrates the fact that there is no perfect treatment for hyperthyroidism. We are restricted to carbimazole or methimazole, I-131 or surgery. The role of propylthiouracil is perhaps restricted to the first 3 months of pregnancy where the marginally better teratogenic potential can be offset against possible hepatotoxicity. Carbimazole rarely produces a lasting remission. The recommendation is that patients who relapse should either have radioiodine or surgery. In most cases this does not happen, especially in children. In many cases, the parents elect to continue with carbimazole indefinitely. This poses a small but unquantified risk of vasculitis, arthritis and hepatotoxicity. There is extensive data on the safety of radioiodine. Yet most parents do not accept it for their children. In patients with a large or multinodular goiter, surgery is the best choice. It has been shown that a surgeon who does many thyroidectomies has a better outcome, irrespective of the age of the patient.

> **Take Home Messages**
> - *Hyperthyroidism in children is a challenge as carbimazole treatment rarely produces a permanent relapse*
> - *As none of the three treatment modalities produce a perfect result, it is important that shared decision making is used to select the treatment. Sometimes parents opt for carbimazole in spite of a recommendation for radioiodine, and after several visits choose I-131 treatment*
> - *No harm has been documented with long term carbimazole but given its side effect profile, some problems are likely in the long term as mentioned in the Discussion. Also if carbimazole is stopped if the patient is ill due to some other reason, hyperthyroidism ensues very quickly and adds to the comorbidity*
> - *It is important to have a dialog with the patient and make a recommendation regarding treatment. The patient may not accept the recommendation and choose something different. If medically feasible, the physician should then go along to implement whatever treatment choices are made.*

SUGGESTED READING

1. Sanyal D, Chatterjee S. Hyperthyroidism in children: treatment outcomes and preferences in Eastern India. Clin Pediatr Endocrinol. 2015;24(2):63-6.
2. Srinivasan S, Misra M. Hyperthyroidism in children. Pediatr Rev. 2015;36(6):239-48.
3. Sundaresh V, Brito JP, Thapa P, et al. Comparative Effectiveness of Treatment Choices for Graves' Hyperthyroidism: A Historical Cohort Study. Thyroid. 2017;27(4):497-505.

CASE 9 | Gynecomastia: An Unusual Initial Presentation of Thyrotoxicosis

Rana Bhattacharjee, Ajitesh Roy, Pradip Mukhopadhyay, Sujoy Ghosh

CASE HISTORY

A 29-year-old male presented with complaint of bilateral painful breast enlargement for 1 month. He had been married with one child aged 5 years. There was a history of generalized weakness, weight loss, and increased appetite. He had no addiction. He was not on any medication. Recently he developed anxiety and premature ejaculation. He was thinly built with normally palpable thyroid without any bruit. He had sinus tachycardia with postural tremor of hands. There is no thyroid associated orbitopathy or dermopathy. Gynecomastia with disk diameter of 3 cm was found. His testicular volume was 25 mL bilaterally. There was no palpable testicular mass. He was well virilized.

The laboratory investigations showed impaired glucose tolerance, normal renal and liver function tests (Table 1).

TABLE 1: Laboratory evaluation.

Tests	Value	Normal range
Free thyroxine	4.1 ng/dL	0.9–1.8
Free triiodothyronine	8.3 pg/mL	2.4–6.6
Thyroid-stimulating hormone	0.03 mIU/mL	0.4–4.0
Testosterone (total)	>915 ng/dL	250–1,600
β-human chorionic gonadotropin	Undetectable	–
Estradiol	105 pg/mL	<50
Luteinizing hormone	9.7 mIU/mL	0.8–7.6
Follicle-stimulating hormone	6.06 mIU/mL	0.7–11.1
Prolactin	15.1 ng/mL	2.5–17

Technetium-99m (Tc-99m) pertechnatate thyroid scan showed diffusely increased uptake. After discussing the treatment options, patient was started on carbimazole. Signs and symptoms of thyrotoxicosis improved within a few weeks. Gynecomastia disappeared within 6 months of starting treatment.

INTRODUCTION

Gynecomastia is a well-recognized manifestation of thyrotoxicosis. However, it is not commonly encountered in clinical practice. Gynecomastia as initial presentation of thyrotoxicosis is extremely unusual.

DISCUSSION

Thyrotoxicosis causes gynecomastia by increasing free estrogen to testosterone ratio by several postulated mechanisms. Thyrotoxicosis increases the hepatic production of sex hormone binding globulin (SHBG). Testosterone binds with SHBG with more affinity in comparison to estradiol. With increasing level of SHBG, free testosterone level decreases. Moreover, thyrotoxicosis causes increased level of luteinizing hormone which stimulates aromatase activity in the Leydig cells. There is also increased conversion of androgen to estrogen by products.

New onset of gynecomastia should be thoroughly evaluated in a middle-aged man. Gynecomastia in this age group is commonly due to medication, renal and liver dysfunction, and various endocrine diseases.

Take Home Messages

- Endocrine evaluation of gynecomastia should be undertaken in appropriate situation
- Gynecomastia is an uncommon, but important manifestation of thyrotoxicosis.

CASE 10: Two Interesting Cases of Raised Thyroid-stimulating Hormone

Sujoy Majumdar

CASE HISTORY

Patient A
- Mrs SB aged 47 years presented with obesity and history of progressive lethargy over last 3 years. She had put on 5 kg in 2 years. She was feeling so lethargic that she was unwilling to embark on any lifestyle measures to reduce her weight. She complained of palpitations and dry, coarse skin and palpitations
- She had previously presented 2 years earlier for a suspected hypothyroidism. A routine thyroid function test showed raised Free T4 8.5 ng/dL (NR: 0.8–2 ng/mL), thyroid stimulating hormone (TSH) 25 µIU/mL (NR: 0.5–4.5 µU/mL). Laboratory error was suspected and patient was asked to repeat test. She lost her faith in the doctor
- She presented to another endocrinologist for a "second opinion". Repeat Free T4 was 7.6 ng/dL and TSH 22.5 µIU/mL
- She was asked to get a CT scan of brain—she was told that she had a "brain tumor"! She got extremely frightened and stopped going to any doctor.

Patient B
- Mr RB aged 25 years, the only son of Mrs. RB, an executive in the software industry presented with a history of progressive lethargy over the last 15 months. He was finding difficult to "remember facts" in his office meetings, an issue he ascribed to job stress. He had put on 10 kg weight in last 1 year, which he felt was due to excessive late night parties and drinks. He also complained of cold intolerance and insomnia.

Clinical and laboratory findings of the two cases are shown in Table 1.

TABLE 1: Clinical and laboratory findings of the two cases (patient A and patient B).

Patient A	Patient B
• BMI: 30	• BMI: 27
• HR: 89 beats/min	• HR: 68 beats/min
• BP: 140/90 mm Hg	• BP: 130/80 mm Hg
• Goiter present but no bruit	• No goiter
• Coarse skin—moist palm	• Skin unremarkable
• Free T4: 7.6 ng/dL	• Free T4: 4.6 ng/dL
• TSH: 16 µIU/mL	• TSH: 12.6 µIU/mL
• Anti-TPO: 35 U/mL	• Anti-TPO: 14 U/mL
• TSH receptor AB: Negative	• TSH receptor AB: Negative

How do you approach the problem?
Free T4 and TSH can be correlated in the following ways (Table 2).
In these two cases the differential diagnoses were:

TABLE 2: Interpretation of lab results of free T4 and TSH.

Free thyroxin	TSH	Interpretation
Normal	Suppressed	• Subclinical hyperthyroidism • Recently treated hyperthyroidism • Nonthyroidal illness (sick euthyroid syndrome) • Drugs: Steroids, dopamine
Raised	Suppressed	• Overt hyperthyroidism
Normal	Raised	• Subclinical hypothyroidism • Poor compliance/malabsorption of levothyroxine in a patient of overt hypothyroidism • Recovery phase of nonthyroidal illness (sick euthyroid syndrome) • Assay interference (TSH autoantibodies, heterophile antibodies) • Drugs: Amiodarone • Adrenal insufficiency
Suppressed	Raised	• Overt hypothyroidism
Suppressed	Suppressed	• Central hypothyroidism (including isolated TSH deficiency) and panhypopituitarism • Nonthyroidal illness (sick euthyroid syndrome)
Raised	Raised	• TSH secreting pituitary adenoma • Resistance to thyroid hormone
Raised	Normal	• Iatrogenic overdose of levothyroxine • Neonatal period

(TSH: thyroid-stimulating hormone)

1. The thyroid-stimulating hormone secreting pituitary adenoma
2. Resistance to thyroid hormone (RTH).

The MRI scan of pituitary was normal in both the patients. The diagnosis was, therefore, resistance to thyroid hormone (TRH).

INTRODUCTION

Thyroid stimulating hormone (TSH) is a glycoprotein hormone synthesized in the thyrotropic cells of the anterior pituitary. It consists of two subunits—α and β. Hormone specificity is conveyed by the β-subunit. Dimerization with α-subunit is necessary for the biological activity of TSH. TSH stimulates the thyroid follicular cells (by binding to a specific TSH receptor) to produce thyroxine (T4) from hydrolysis of thyroglobulin by lysosomal proteases. In plasma, T4 is largely bound to thyroxine binding globulin (TBG) (approximately 75%) and to a lesser extent to transthyretin (approximately 10%) and albumin (approximately 15%), leaving around 0.02% as Free T4. Free T4 is the metabolically active T4. Free T4 levels in blood regulate TSH levels by a negative feedback mechanism. On the whole elevated TSH >5.0 μU/mL indicates primary hypothyroidism, while a TSH <0.1 μU/mL indicates hyperthyroidism.

T4 is converted to T3 by the deiodinase enzymes and the principal effects of T3 are conveyed through a nuclear thyroid receptor (TR). In humans there are two homologous TRs-α and β. There can be a resistance to either of these and this can bring about bizarre blood results of Free T4 and TSH.

DISCUSSION

Majority of patients of RTH have a mutation in the *TR-β* gene that interferes with the capacity of that receptor to respond normally to T3 by reducing T3 binding affinity (generalized resistance). A minority may have hyperthyroidism if more severe resistance in the hypothalamic region (pituitary resistance). Mutant TR-β complexes can interfere with the functioning of the three normal TR expressing genes, producing a pattern termed dominant negative inhibition with an autosomal dominant pattern. Resistance to thyroid hormone action at the level of pituitary and hypothalamus due to abnormal TR-β signaling gives rise to the classical biochemical picture of raised TSH and Free T4 and T3.

The frequency of the condition is 1:40,000–50,000 live births and a little more than 1,000 individuals have been described till date in >350 families.

Goiter is present in two-thirds of patients. Palpitation due to sinus tachycardia (atrial fibrillation in a few cases) is more common than bradycardia. Other clinical features include a raised basal metabolic rate and reduced bone mineral density. Dyslipidemia is also noted in a certain proportion of patients.

When presenting for the first time in childhood and adolescence, the classical features are failure to thrive, hyperphagia and recurrent infections of ear nose and throat. Neuropsychological deficiencies including increased prevalence of attention deficit hyperactivity disorder (ADHD) are also prevalent. Deafness due to lack of development in the hearing mechanism. Mixture of symptoms differs within the same family.

Definitive diagnosis requires sequencing of the *TR-β* gene—found in 90% individuals with the diagnosis.

Differentiating a TR-β TRH from TSHoma is primarily done by an MRI. Other tests like TRH (thyrotropin release hormone) stimulation test and LT3 suppression test are helpful but difficult to do in Indian settings.

Treatment is essentially symptomatic like β-blockers for palpitation, statins for dyslipidemia. T3 analog like TRIAC (triiodothyroacetic acid) has been shown to lower T4, T3 and TSH in some patients.

Take Home Message

- *All patients should not be diagnosed as having hypothyroidism simply on the basis of a single raised TSH. The test should be repeated along with Free T4 to confirm the diagnosis of hypothyroidism. In the presence of RTH treatment with thyroid hormone replacement is disastrous.*

SUGGESTED READING

1. Gurnell M, Visser T, Beck-Peccoz P, et al. Resistance to Thyroid Hormone. In: Jameson JI, De Groot LJ (Eds). Endocrinology, 7th Edition. Philadelphia: Saunders; 2015. pp. 1649-65.
2. Moran C, Agostini M, Visser WE, et al. Resistance to thyroid hormone caused by a mutation in the thyroid hormone receptor TRα1 and TRα2; clinical, biochemical and genetic analysis of three related patients. Lancet Diabetes Endocrinol. 2014;2:619-26.

INDEX

Page numbers followed by *b* refer to box, *f* refer to figure, *t* refer to table and *fc* refer to flowchart.

A

Abdomen
    CT scan of 15*f*
    ultrasonography of 18
Abscess 45
Acanthosis nigricans 28, 121*f*
Acetylcholinesterase inhibitor test 153
Achalasia 14
    cardia 13*f*, 83
Acidosis, systemic 19
Addison's disease 11, 68
Adenoma, unilateral 8
Adrenal function, evaluation of 105*t*
Adrenal glands
    bilateral 2*f*
    normal 8*f*
Adrenal histoplasmosis 1
    treatment of 2
Adrenal hyperplasia
    bilateral 8, 9*f*
    unilateral primary 8
Adrenal incidentaloma 4
Adrenal insufficiency 16, 138
    evolving primary 14
    severity of 2
Adrenal tuberculosis 16
Adrenal-dependent causes 7
Adrenocortical insufficiency 124
Alacrima 13*f*, 14
Alanine aminotransferase 117
Albumin 11, 30, 169
    creatinine 50
    low 20
    normal 20
Albuminuria, absence of 37
Aldosteronism, primary 9
Alkaline phosphatase 21, 30
    bone-specific 20
Alkaline urine, presence of 19
Allgrove's syndrome 14
Amenorrhea, etiology of 118
Amitriptyline 77
Amyloidosis 84
Analgesia 65
Androgen deprivation therapy 58
Angioplasty with stenting 91*f*
Angiotensin-converting enzyme 82
Angular cheilitis 14
Anion gap 18
Ankle foot orthosis 89*f*
Anorexia 11
Antibiotics, systemic 78
Anticholinesterase medications 153
Anti-glutamic acid decarboxylase 24
Antihyperglycemic agents 50
Antihypertensive medications 6
Antinuclear antibody 18
Antipsychotics 58
Antiretroviral therapy 58
Anti-thyroid peroxidase 108
Antitubercular therapy 16
Anxiety 124
Aorta, coarctation of 6
Appetite, increased 100
Arginine vasopressin 113
Arthritis 166
    debilitating 136
Ascites 51
Aspartate aminotransferase 117
Asymptomatic disease 133
Atherosclerotic cardiovascular disease 48, 49
Atrial fibrillation 164, 170
    paroxysmal 163
Atrophic pancreas 62
Autistic behavior 109
Autoimmune adrenal insufficiency 152
Autoimmune diabetes 29, 68
    adults, late onset 29
Autoimmune disease 12, 101, 104, 124
Autoimmune hypophysitis 137
Autoimmune polyendocrine syndrome 12
Autoimmune regulator 12
Autoimmune thyroid disease 152, 153
Autonomic nervous system abnormalities 14
Azoospermia 66
    persistent 66
    simulates obstructive 66

B

Balloon dilatation 91, 92*f*
Barefoot walking, history of 94
Behavioral disorder 107

Bilirubin 11
   total 30, 60
Biochemistry, baseline 60*t*
Biothesiometer 97*f*
Bleeding, regular cyclic 26
Blood
   biochemistry 78
   cell count 45
   routine 11
   sodium concentration 112
   transfusions 25
Blood glucose
   chart 40*t*
   fasting 38
   increase 58, 58*t*
   less 123
   level 31*t*
   low 124
Blood pressure 11, 138
   systolic 67
   visit-to-visit systolic 37
Blood sugar 39, 40
   high 40
Body mass index 117, 123
   low 60
Body weight, changes in 101*t*
Brachial index 90
Breast cancer 104
Brown tumors 128, 132

C

Calcium
   channel 77
   supplementation 23
Cancer death, cause of 62
Capillary blood glucose reading 71*t*
Carbimazole 164, 165
Cardinal symptoms 11
Cardiovascular disease 49
Carpal tunnel syndrome 74, 136
Celiac disease 68
Cell-mediated immunity 16
Cellulitis 45, 65, 85
   differential diagnosis of 87
   mimic in diabetes 44
Central venous sinus thrombosis 110, 111
Charcot foot, diagnosis of 87
Charcot's arthropathy 87
Charcot's foot 86
Charcot's joint 84
   acute 84
Charcot's neuro-osteoarthropathy 85
   demonstrates 85
Charcot's osteoarthropathy 87
Charcot-Marie-Tooth disease 84
Chills 27
Cholangiopancreatography, magnetic resonance 61*f*

Cholesterol 50
Common bile duct, dilatation of 61*f*
Conductance regulator, transmembrane 66
Confusional state, acute 129
   causes of 132*b*
Conjunctival congestion 150*f*
Conjunctival edema 150*f*
Consciousness, loss of 142
Coronary artery bypass 47
Cortical cells, hypertrophy of 16
Corticotropin 140
Cough 27
Coxsackievirus infection 71
C-peptide level, fasting 27
C-reactive protein 45, 158
Creatine phosphokinase 64
Creatinine 11, 21, 30, 100
   kinase 45
Crohn's disease 101
Cryptococcosis 2
Cushing's syndrome 7
Cushingoid appearance 118
Cystic fibrosis 66
   related diabetes 66
Cystinosis 22
Cytomegalovirus infection 2

D

Deep tendon reflexes 156
Deep venous thrombosis 45, 65
Deferasirox 23
Dehydration
   absence of 111
   severe 78
Delusional symptoms 30
Dementia care 32
Diabetes 27, 46, 135
   and breast 41
   and heart failure 48
   and hypogonadism 26
   care 32
   complication of 46, 63
   double 69, 71
   duration of 77
   family history of 68
   hand syndrome, tropical 34
   in adult, late onset 67
   ketosis prone 29
   management 28
   optimize 26
   risk factors of 25
   systems of 68
Diabetes mellitus 25, 32, 38, 72, 84, 105
   long-standing 44, 64
   male hypertensive with 134
   management of type 2 54, 58
   type 1 25, 33, 41, 64, 68, 71, 111, 152
   type 2 25, 37, 42, 44, 50, 54, 57, 69, 75, 79, 90, 96, 110, 120, 127, 129, 136

Diabetic cardiomyopathy 48
Diabetic complications 37
Diabetic foot
   infection 93, 94
   infection, severe 94
   neuropathic 96
   osteomyelitis 94
Diabetic ketoacidosis 27, 28, 28f, 132
   diagnosis of 38, 78
   management of 38
   manifestation of 77
Diabetic kidney disease 94
Diabetic lumbosacral plexopathy 65
Diabetic mastopathy 41
   diagnosis of 43t
Diabetic muscle infarction 44
Diabetic myonecrosis 44, 45
   diagnosis of 44
   differential diagnosis of 45t
Diabetic nephropathy, advanced 35
Diabetic neuropathy 75, 77
Diabetic peripheral neuropathy 96
Diabetic retinopathy 35
   evidence of 36f
Diabetic truncal radiculoneuropathy 75
Dipeptidyl peptidase-4 49
Disability, learning 32
Distended gastric shadow 78f
Distension 78
Dizziness, symptoms of 112
Dorsalis pedis 94
Duloxetine 77
Dysglycemia, cases of 122
Dyslipidemia 170
Dysmorphic facial features 109
Dysuria 27

E

Eating disorder 33
Echogenicities 65
Ectopic adenomas 132
Edema 51
Ejaculation, premature 166
Ejection fraction 46
   preserved 48, 51
   regional 48
Elbow joints 134
Electrolytes 138
Electromyography, single-fiber 153
Empagliflozin 47
Endocrine 26, 132
   conditions 5
   emergency 78
Endocrinology consultation 138
Endoscopic fundoplication 83
End-systolic volumes 48
Eosinophilia 11
Erythrocyte sedimentation rate 23, 34, 45, 64, 70

Esophageal manometry 13
Estrogen 101
Estrogen replacement 24f
   therapy 101
Euthyroidism, restoration of 150
Excisional biopsy, treatment with 43
Extraocular muscle
   infiltration of 153
   motility 153
Eyeballs, enlarging 100

F

Facial hirsutism 116
Factitious 124
Fanconi's syndrome 20
Fatty acid oxidation 78
Febuxostat 47
Femoral epiphyseal dysgenesis 21f
Femur, left 18f
Fever 27
   low grade 78
Fibrocalculus pancreatic diabetes 60, 66
Flatbush diabetes mellitus 28
Fleshy nose 74
Fluorine-labeled fluorodeoxyglucose 125
Fluoroquinolones 123
Folic acid 23
Follicle-stimulating hormone 24, 25, 66, 100, 108, 117, 142, 143
Foot
   temperature assessment 88f
   ulcers, recurrent 94
Forefoot 86
Fragile X syndrome 109, 109t
Fringe nerve damage 86
Fungal infections 2

G

Gabapentin 77
Gap metabolic acidosis 78
Gastric dilatation, acute 77
   causes of 79
Gastroesophageal reflux 83
Gastrointestinal blood flow 113
Gastrointestinal endoscopy 21
   upper 82
Gastroparesis, severe 79
Genetic insulin resistance 25
Genu valgum deformity 21f
Gestational thyrotoxicosis 154, 155
Giant cell granuloma 127f
Gingival mass 127f
Glargine 47
Glimepiride 106
Globulin 11, 30
Glomerular filtration rate 50
   estimated 49

Glomerulosclerosis 36
Glossitis 14
Glucagon-like peptide-1 receptor agonist 49
Glucocorticoid 58, 164
   remediable aldosteronism 8
Glucosamine 59
Glucose
   monitoring system
      continuous 80
      helped 79
   parameters, stable 39t
   values, postprandial 80
Glucosuria 20
Glutamic acid decarboxylase 28, 29
Glycemia 134
Glycemic control 63, 66, 79
   deterioration of 67
   poor 30t
Glycosylated hemoglobin 23, 25, 27t, 34t, 49f, 76, 80
Glycosylation end products 42
Gonadotropin 140
   releasing hormone 143
Gout 85, 87
Graves' disease 151, 154, 155, 164
   diagnosis of 101, 152
Graves' ophthalmopathy, sign of 152
Growth hormone 140
   deficiency 25, 106
   excessive 135
   secreting pituitary macroadenoma 74
Gynecomastia 166, 167
   bilateral 102f

H

Hair
   on axilla, absent 102f
   on body, absent 102f
   on face, absent 102f
Headache 74, 142
   symptoms of 112
Healing after amputation 92f
Heart failure 46, 48, 51
   hospitalization for 50, 51
   prevention of 52t
   risk of 48
   symptoms of 52t
Hematoma 65
Hematuria 5
Hemoglobin 13, 23, 34, 60
   abnormal 81
   case of 23
   E-beta thalassemia 23, 25
Hemorrhagic infarct, subacute 110f
Hepatitis C antibodies 103
Hepatotoxicity 166
Hexosamine 59
Hip joint, X-ray of 21f
Hirsutism 121f

Histoplasma 2
Histoplasmosis 2
Hormone
   adrenocorticotropic 14, 117, 142
   therapy 105
Hot flashes in men 136, 137
Human chorionic gonadotropin 154
Human immunodeficiency virus 2, 117
Human leukocyte antigen 28, 29
Hungry bone syndrome 133
Hydrocortisone 10, 11
Hydroxytryptophan 125
Hyperactivity disorder, attention deficit 170
Hyperaldosteronism, primary 6
Hypercalcemia 62, 128
   causes of 130b
Hyperglycemia
   incidence of 58
   treatment algorithm 49f
   uncontrolled 134
Hyperglycemic state, unexplained 57
Hypergonadotropic hypogonadism 103
Hyperhidrosis 136
Hyperparathyroidism, primary 127
Hyperphagia, symptoms of 106
Hyperplasia, causes 148
Hyperprolactinemia 143
Hypertension 5, 9, 48, 63, 129, 136
   causes 5
      for secondary 5b
   endocrine causes of 7b
   paroxysmal 4
   presence of 4
   systemic 127
Hyperthyroid child 165
Hyperthyroidism 100, 101
Hypertrichosis 147f
Hypertriglyceridemia 110, 111
Hypocalcemia, biochemical 133
Hypochromic anemia, mild microcytic 20
Hypoechoic mass 42
Hypoglycemia 11, 123, 146
   attack 40
   cases of 125t
   lower risk of 55
   symptoms of 124
   workup for 123, 124
Hypogonadism 106
   correction of 25
Hypogonadotropic hypogonadism 25
Hypokalemia 11, 19, 20, 157
Hypokalemic paralysis 157
Hypokalemic periodic paralysis, familial 156, 156t
Hypokinesia 46
   global 47f
Hyponatremia 10, 11, 113fc
   epidemiology of exercise-associated 112
   exercise-associated 112

management of exercise-associated 114*t*
prevention of exercise-associated 114
Hypoparathyroidism 26
Hypophosphatemia 20
Hypophysitis, clinical suspicion of 138
Hypopituitarism 124, 140
Hypotension 78
Hypothalamic–pituitary–gonadal axis 143*f*
Hypothalamo-pituitary region 147*f*
Hypothyroid 163
Hypothyroidism 129, 131
   and infection 52
   clinical stigma of 146*f*
   primary 148
   secondary 144

I

Immunofluorescent antinuclear antibody 34, 35
Infected hand, diabetic with 33
Infection, acute 27
Inflammatory cells 2*f*
Infrared thermometer, handheld 87
Inherited developmental disability, cause of 109
Insensate foot 87
Insulin 123, 150
   action 79
   infusion 78
   injection 40
   levels of 125
   pen devices 82
   regimen 28
   regular 47
   resistance, signs of 28
   therapy, basal-bolus 24
Insulinoma 124
   imaging for 124
   tumors-like 124
Intellectual disability 109
Interferon-α 58
Interleukin 113
Intramuscular injection 152
Intrathyroidal vascularity 152
Intravascular coagulation, disseminated 140
Intravascular hemolysis 140
Intravenous
   fluids 69, 78
   potassium 78
Irritation 85
Ischemic cardiomyopathy 48
Ischemic diabetic foot 90
Islet cell autoimmunity 29
Islet tyrosine phosphatase 2 antibodies 24, 29
Isotonic saline 114

J

Jaundice, obstructive 62
Juvenile rheumatoid arthritis 101

K

Kayser-Fleischer ring 21*f*
Ketoacidosis, absence of 111
Ketosis-prone diabetes, classification of 29*t*
Kidney
   disease, chronic 49
   injury in dengue, acute 71
Klebsiella pneumonia 34
Knee
   joints 134
   prosthesis, below 95*f*
Köbberling type 118

L

Lacrimal gland, absent 13*f*
Langerhans, islets of 71
Left ankle and foot 84
Left foot
   acute charcot of 85*f*
   swollen 87*f*
Left leg, deep skin ulcers on 103*f*
Left thumb
   gangrene in 33*f*, 34*f*
   ulceration in 33*f*
Leprosy 84
Leucocyte count, total 23, 34, 60, 158
Lid-edema 150*f*
Lip biopsy specimens 18*f*
Lipoatrophy 118
Lipodystrophy 118
   acquired
      generalized 118
      partial 118
   familial partial 115, 118
Lipoprotein
   high-density 105, 106, 117
   low-density 50, 105, 106
Liquid chromatography, high performance 81
Liver
   dysfunction 27, 52
   function test 34, 50, 105, 106
Lowe's syndrome 22
Lower jaw, brown tumor of 127
Lower limb amputations 95
Lumbar hernia 76*f*
Lumbar swelling, left-sided 76*f*
Lumpectomy 41
Luteinizing hormone 24, 25, 66, 100, 105, 108, 117, 139, 142, 143
Lymphadenopathy 15
Lymphocytic infiltration 42*f*, 156
Lymphocytic mastitis 41

M

Macroglossia 73, 74, 134, 135*f*
Macroorchidism 109
   boy with 107

Macroprolactinoma 143
Male infertility, treatable cause of 142
Malnutrition 78
Mandibular mass, left 128f
McCune-Albright syndrome 108
Mental retardation 109
  mild 106
Metabolic abnormalities 79
Metabolic acidosis 19, 78
Metabolic disorders 118
Metabolic syndrome 68, 104
Metatarsal heads 86
Metatarsophalangeal joints 84
Metformin 106
Methimazole 165
Microvascular dysfunction 48
Mineralocorticoid receptor 6
Monofilament test 97f
Mortality, associated 51
Mosaic Klinefelter syndrome 103
Mucous membranes 13
Muscle
  abscess 65
  atrophy 76f
  right vastus anterior 63f
  rupture 65
  weakness 19, 157fc
Musculoskeletal abnormality 146
Myasthenia gravis 153
Myasthenic symptoms 153
Mycobacterium tuberculosis 16
Myonecrosis 63
Myxedema coma 158, 160, 161t

N

Narcotics 65
Nausea 78
  symptoms of 112
Necrotizing fasciitis 45, 65
Neostigmine 152f
  before 152f
  minutes after 152f
Nephrocalcinosis 19
  right-sided 18f
Nephrolithiasis 19, 132
Nephropathy 44, 55
Nerve stimulation test, repetitive 152
Neuroglycopenic symptoms 124
Neuro-osteoarthropathy 85
Neuropathic assessment 97
Neuropathic joints 84
Neuropathic osteoarthropathy 86
Neuropathic pain 77
Neuropathic ulcers 97
Neuropathy 44, 55
Neuropsychiatric symptoms 128
Neutrophil 11
Nonhealing ulcers 94

Nonsteroidal anti-inflammatory drugs 113
Nonstructural protein 1 70
Noradrenaline reuptake inhibitors 77
Normoglycemia, spite of 81
Nuclear thyroid receptor 170

O

Obesity 106
Ocular myasthenia gravis 151, 152
Oligomenorrhea 120
Ophthalmoplegia 152, 153
Oral antidiabetic agents 63, 71
Oral calcium, long-term 133
Oral hypoglycemic agents 28
Organic cardiac lesions 103
Osteitis fibrosa cystic 132
Osteomyelitis 85-87
  joint 84
Osteoporosis 128
Ovaries 120

P

Pancreas 123, 124
Pancreatic adenocarcinoma 60
Pancreatic beta cells 125
Pancreatic cancer, risk of 62
Pancreatic duct, course of main 61f
Pancreatic dysfunction 66
Pancreatitis 128
  chronic 62
  tropical calcific 62
Paraneoplastic syndromes 124
Parathyroid
  adenoma 131f
  dependent causes 7
Parathyroidectomy 133
  right inferior 127
Parkinsonism 129
Pedal pulses, palpation of 91f
Peripheral artery disease 90, 94
Peripheral neuropathy 94, 97
Peripheral pulses 94
Peripheral vascular disease 55
Pernicious anemia 152
Pertechnetate thyroid 156
Pheochromocytoma without hypertension 3
Phosphorus 17
Pituitary 134
  damage 140
  dependent causes 7
  dysfunction 25, 141
  failure, chronic 141
  gland 138f
  hyperplasia
    diffuse 147f
    secondary 148
  hypofunction 137

macroadenoma 108, 135f
mass 148
resistance 170
thyrotrophic cells 148
Plasma
  aldosterone concentration 6
  glucose
    fasting 24, 27, 34, 64, 100, 105, 106, 110, 142
    postprandial 27, 34, 64, 105, 106
  osmolality 138
  renin activity 6
Polyarthralgia, complaints of 134
Polycystic ovarian syndrome 115, 118, 120, 121
  diagnosis of 115
Polyethylene glycol 142
Polysomnogram 107
Polyurethane-coated fiberglass 97
Post-amputation 91f
  healed stump 95f
Postmenopausal ladies 17
Post-pacemaker implantation 10
Potassium 11, 13, 21, 105
Prader orchidometer beads 108
Pregabalin 77
Pregnancy hormones 155
Proinsulin 125t
Prolactin 100, 140, 148
Prolactinoma 142
  effects of 143fc
Proptosis eye ball 150f
Propylthiouracil, role of 165
Protein, total 11, 30
Pseudofracture 17
Pseudomonas aeruginosa 34
Psoriasis 101
Psychiatric illnesses 31
Puberty
  delayed 106
  girl with delayed 23
Pulse generator 10
Pyomyositis, tropical 65
Pyuria 5

R

Radioiodine therapy 157
Red blood cells 117
Refractory rickets 20, 21
Rehydration drinks 114
Renal biopsy 37
Renal dysfunction 27
Renal failure, develop 140
Renal functions, normal 20
Renal parenchymal disease 5
Renal stones 128
Renal tubular acidosis 19
  distal 17
Retinopathy 37, 44, 55
Rheumatoid joint pain 85
Rickets in children, cause of 22
Rigorous glycemic control 46

S

Salicylates 123
Salivary glands, minor 18f
Salt, pinch of 112
Schirmer's test 18
Seborrhea 134
Septic joint pain 85
Septic shock 123
Serotonin 77
Serum 78
  amylase 11
  bicarbonate 18
  calcium 17, 132, 133
  C-receptive protein 86
  electrolytes 124
  glutamic-oxaloacetic transaminase 23, 70
  glutamic-pyruvic transaminase 23, 70, 160
  lipase 11
  phosphate 21
  potassium 18
  triglyceride level, high 110
Sex hormone binding globulin 167
Shakiness 124
Short stature 14
Sinus
  tachycardia 47f, 170
  tract 86
Sjögren's syndrome 19
Sleep apnea
  obstructive 5, 107
  syndrome 136
Snake bite 140
Sodium 11, 105
  supplements 114
Somatostatin analogs 58
Spastic dysarthria 21
Splenectomy 23
Sports medicine community 112
Staphylococcus aureus 34
Statin 58
  postdischarge 47
Steatorrhea
  in adolescence 62
  in childhood 62
Steroid replacement therapy 138
Stomach, barium meal of 82f
Stress, repetitive 87
Stroke 55
Subcutaneous fat 115
  reduced 116f
Subcutaneous insulin, multi-dose 47
Subtrochanteric fracture 18f
  left-sided 17f
Sulfonylureas 123
Sweating 124
Symptomatic disease, treatment for 133
Syringomyelia 84

T

Tachycardia 78, 124
Temper tantrums 104, 106
Testes, localize 105
Tetracosactrin, injection 15
Thalassemia care 26
Thermoregulatory dysfunction 161
Thiazide diuretics 58
Thrombocytopenic purpura, idiopathic 101
Thrombophlebitis 65
Thyroglobulin 169
Thyroid 101, 146
   autoantibodies 101
   autoimmunity 101
   binding globulin 154
   dependent causes 7
   disorder 124
     treatment of 152
   dysfunction 101
     management of 153
   function 101t
     creatinine normal 27
     in pregnancy 154
     tests 15, 100, 156
   hormone 140
     replacement 148
   ophthalmopathy 149
   stimulating hormone 24, 101, 105, 106, 108, 117, 139, 142, 148, 159, 169
     cases of 168
Thyroidectomy 157
Thyroiditis 156, 162
   factitia 164
   painless 156
   subacute 163, 163f
Thyrotoxic periodic paralysis 156, 156t, 157f
Thyrotoxic symptoms 152
Thyrotoxicosis 155, 166
   diagnosed in pregnancy, differential diagnosis of 154
   in pregnancy, management of 155
Thyrotropic cells 169
Thyrotropin release hormone 148, 170
Thyroxine 140, 145, 169
   binding globulin 169
   dose of 11
   free 24, 101
   low 148
   replacement 148
   surreptitious intake of 164
Tibial artery, posterior 84
Toes, blackening of 90f
Total contact cast 87, 88, 89f
Transabdominal ultrasound 125
Transaminases, normal 20
Trans-sphenoidal pituitary surgery 136
Transthyretin 169
Trauma fracture, low 17
Tricyclic antidepressants, efficacies of 77
Triglycerides 105, 106
Triiodothyroacetic acid 170
Triiodothyronine, free 101
Triple A syndrome 13, 14
Truncal radiculoneuropathy 77
Tuberculosis 16
Tubular functions, derangement of 22
Turner's syndrome 100, 100f, 101
Tyrosine
   kinase inhibitors 58
   phosphatase 2 antibodies 28
Tyrosinemia 22

U

Ulcer 86
   debridement of 97
Undescended testes, bilateral 106
Urea 11, 30
Uric acid 30
Urinary
   sulfonylurea 125t
   tract infections 5
Urine
   anion gap 18
   ketones 78

V

Vas deferens, congenital absence of both 66
Vascular dementia, diagnosis of 129
Vasculitis, risk of 166
Vein thrombosis, profound 85
Venous thromboembolism 111
Vision, blurring of 142
Visual field defects 74
Vitamin D
   concentrations 17
   deficiency of 22, 132
   doses of 20
   resistant rickets 22
Vitiligo 101, 124
Vomiting 78

W

Whipple's triad 124
Wilson's disease 20-22
Wound
   closure 98f
   ultrasonic debridement of 92f
Wrist joints 134

X

X chromosome 101

Y

Yeast cells, small 2f

Cipla

Cordially Invites all the Delegates of

IDEACON – 2019
Kolkata

BASAGLAR®
Insulin Glargine I.P. Solution for Injection 100 U/mL

VYSOV-M®
Vildagliptin 50 mg + Metformin HCl 500/1000 mg Tablets

PROMINAD®
Canagliflozin 100 mg Tablets

Cipla

In management of type 2 diabetes

Vysov - M®

Vildagliptin 50 mg + Metformin HCl 500 mg/1000 mg Tablets

SMOOTH CONTROL. SMOOTH LIFE.

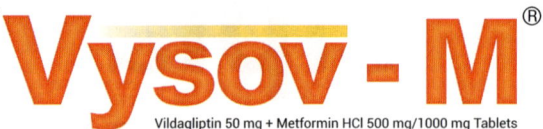

VERIFY
Vildagliptin **E**fficacy in combination with
metfo**R**min **F**or earl**Y** treatment of type 2 diabetes

First study to investigate the long-term clinical benefits of early (HbA1C 6.5-7.5%) dual combination treatment versus the standard-of-care metformin monotherapy followed by addition of oral antihyperglycaemic agent[1]

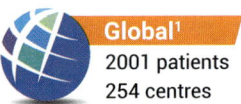

Global[1]
2001 patients
254 centres

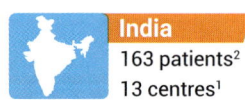

India
163 patients[2]
13 centres[1]

PATIENT CHARACTERISTICS AT BASELINE[1]

Mean HbA1C	Median diabetes duration	Mean BMI
6.9%	3.4 months	31.1 kg/m²

Study Design[3]

			Period 1‡	Period 2§	Period 3	
†Metformin 500 mg/day	Metformin 1000 mg/day	Metformin 1500 mg/day	Metformin upto 1000 mg twice daily + Vildagliptin 50 mg bid	Metformin upto 1000 mg twice daily + Vildagliptin 50 mg bid		+ (Basal) insulin*
Screening 2 weeks	Run-in 3 weeks n ~ 2000	Randomisation	HbA1C ≥ 7.0% (twice)		At investigator discretion	
			Metformin upto 1000 mg twice daily + placebo bid	Metformin upto 1000 mg twice daily + Vildagliptin 50 mg bid		+ (Basal) insulin*

Visit every 3 monthly

Day 1 ———————————————————————— 5 years

Results to be declared during EASD 2019 (September)

Smooth control refers to effective glycaemic control (refer the published article for reductions in HbA1C and other parameters) Smooth life refers to reduced incidence of adverse events during study period (refer the published article for incidence of adverse events) BMI: Body Mass Index, EASD: European Association for the Study of Diabetes

References: • Insulin initiation according to local guidelines. † Metformin dose can be adjusted in the first 4 weeks of randomisation up to 2000 mg, or the maximal tolerated dose. No adjustment is allowed afterwards ‡ Period duration can differ between the two treatments. The end of period 1 is defined by the day when the patient will receive a new Vildagliptin medication packs because of HbA1c ≥ 53 mmol/mol (7.0%) measured at two consecutive scheduled visits. § Participants in both arms will receive Vildagliptin in a medication pack designed differently from the Vildagliptin/placebo packs used in period 1. 1. Matthews DR et. al., Diabet Med. 2018 Dec 21. 2. Mohan V, et al. Oral Presentations, Abstract 15; DiabetesIndia February 28 - March 3, 2019 (Jaipur). 3. Del Prato S, et al. Diabet Med. 2014 Oct;31(10):1178-84.

Abridged Prescribing Information: VYSOV-M® Presentation: Tablets containing vildagliptin/metformin hydrochloride fixed dose combination: 50 mg/500 mg, 50 mg/1,000 mg. Indication: • Vysov M is indicated as an adjunct to diet and exercise to improve glycaemic control in patients with type 2 diabetes mellitus (T2DM) whose diabetes is not adequately controlled on metformin hydrochloride or vildagliptin alone or who are already treated with the combination of vildagliptin and metformin hydrochloride, as separate tablets. • Vysov M is indicated in combination with a sulphonylurea (i.e., triple combination therapy) as an adjunct to diet and exercise in patients inadequately controlled with vildagliptin and a sulphonylurea. • Vysov M is indicated in combination with insulin (i.e., triple combination therapy) as an adjunct to diet and exercise to improve glycaemic control in patients when stable dose of insulin and metformin alone do not provide adequate glycaemic control. • Vysov M is also indicated for the treatment of type 2 diabetes mellitus having HbA1C > 8% where diabetes is not adequately controlled by diet and exercise alone. Dosage and administration: • Do not exceed the maximum recommended daily dose of vildagliptin (100 mg). • Should be given with meals. • Adults: Starting dose for patients inadequately controlled on vildagliptin or metformin hydrochloride monotherapy: 50 mg/500mg twice daily and gradually titrated after assessing the adequacy of therapeutic response. • Starting dose for patients switching from combination therapy of vildagliptin plus metformin hydrochloride as separate tablets: 50 mg/500 mg, 50 mg/1,000 mg bid based on the dose of vildagliptin or metformin already being taken. • Starting dose for treatment-naive patients: May be initiated at 50 mg/500 mg daily and gradually titrated to a maximum dose of 50 mg/1,000 mg bid after assessing the adequacy of therapeutic response. • Use in combination with a sulphonylurea or with insulin: The dose of Vysov M should provide vildagliptin dosed as 50 mg twice daily (100 mg total daily dose) and a dose of metformin similar to the dose already being taken. • Renal impairment: Dosage adjustment may be required in patients with creatinine clearance between 30 and 90 ml/min. • Geriatric patients: Dosage should be adjusted based on renal function. • Children (under 18 years of age): Not recommended. Contraindications: • Known hypersensitivity to vildagliptin or metformin hydrochloride or to any of the excipients. • Patients with creatinine clearance <30 ml/min • Congestive heart failure. • Acute or chronic metabolic acidosis including lactic acidosis or diabetic ketoacidosis with or without coma • Should be temporarily discontinued in patients undergoing radiologic studies involving intravascular administration of iodinated contrast materials. Warnings and precautions: • Risk of lactic acidosis. • Monitoring of renal function before treatment initiation and regularly thereafter. • Caution with concomitant use of medications that may affect renal function or metformin hydrochloride disposition. • Vysov M should be temporarily discontinued in patients undergoing radiologic studies involving intravascular administration of iodinated contrast materials. • Discontinue treatment in case of hypoxaemia. • Temporary discontinuation in patients undergoing surgical procedure. • Excessive alcohol intake to be avoided. • Not recommended in patients with hepatic impairment including patients with a pre-treatment ALT or AST >2.5x the upper limit of normal. Liver function tests (LFT) to be performed prior to treatment initiation, at three-month intervals during the first year and periodically thereafter. Withdrawal of therapy with Vysov M recommended if an increase in ALT or AST of 3x upper limit normal or greater persist. Following withdrawal of treatment with Vysov M and LFT normalisation, treatment with Vysov M should not be reinitiated. • Risk of decreased vitamin B12 serum levels. • Should not be used in patients with type 1 diabetes or for the treatment of diabetic ketoacidosis. • Risk of hypoglycaemia. • May be temporarily withheld in case of loss of glycemic control. • Elderly patients' renal function should be assessed more frequently. • Not recommended in paediatric patients. Women of child-bearing potential, pregnancy: Should not be used in pregnancy unless the potential benefit justifies the potential risk to the foetus. Breastfeeding: Should not be used during breastfeeding. Adverse reactions: Vildagliptin: Rare cases of hepatic dysfunction (including hepatitis). Vildagliptin monotherapy – Common: Dizziness – Uncommon: Headache, constipation, oedema peripheral. • Metformin monotherapy – Very common: Loss of appetite, flatulence, nausea, vomiting, diarrhoea, abdominal pain. Common: Dysgeusia. Very rare: Lactic acidosis, hepatitis, skin reactions such as erythema, pruritus and urticaria, decrease of vitamin B12 absorption, liver function test abnormalities. • Other effects with combination of vildagliptin and metformin – Common: Tremor, dizziness, headache. • Other effects with combination of vildagliptin and metformin with insulin – Common: Headache, nausea, gastroesophageal reflux disease, chills, blood glucose decreased – Uncommon: Diarrhoea, flatulence. • Other effects with combination of vildagliptin and metformin with a sulphonylurea – Common: Dizziness, tremor, asthenia, hypoglycaemia, hyperhidrosis. • Post-marketing experience: – Rare: Hepatitis (reversible upon drug discontinuation). • Uncommon: Urticaria, bullous and exfoliative skin lesions including bullous pemphigoid, pancreatitis, arthralgia, sometimes severe. Interactions: • Interactions with vildagliptin: Low potential for drug interactions, no clinically relevant interactions with other oral antidiabetics (glibenclamide, pioglitazone, metformin), amlodipine, digoxin, ramipril, simvastatin, valsartan or warfarin were observed after co-administration with vildagliptin. • Interactions with metformin hydrochloride: Furosemide, nifedipine, cationic drugs, drugs tending to produce hypoglycaemia, alcohol. Packs: Box containing 6 strips of 10 tablets each. Note: Before prescribing, consult full prescribing information available from Cipla Ltd. Cipla House, Peninsula Business Park, Ganpatrao Kadam Marg, Lower Parel, Mumbai - 400 013, India. Website: www.cipla.com. India BSS dtd 12 Jan 17 corrected on 29 May 17 based on international BSS dtd 28 Nov 16, effective from 29 May 17.

"The views, opinions, ideas etc expressed therein are solely that of the author. Novartis does not certify the accuracy, completeness, currency of any information and shall not be responsible or in anyway liable for any errors, omissions or inaccuracies in such information. Novartis is not liable to you in any manner whatsoever for any decision made or action or non-action taken by you in reliance upon the information provided. Novartis does not recommend the use of its products in unapproved indications and recommends to refer to complete prescribing information prior to using any of the Novartis products."
"Issued in scientific service to medical professionals"

For any further information, please contact:

Cipla

Cipla Ltd. Regd. Office: Cipla House, Peninsula Business Park, Ganpatrao Kadam Marg, Lower Parel, Mumbai - 400013, India. Website: www.cipla.com